Freud's Theory and Its Use in
Literary and Cultural Studies

Studies in German Literature, Linguistics, and Culture

Edited by James Hardin
(*South Carolina*)

Freud's Theory and Its Use in Literary and Cultural Studies

AN INTRODUCTION

Henk de Berg

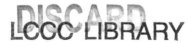
CAMDEN HOUSE

First published 2003
by Camden House

Camden House is an imprint of Boydell & Brewer Inc.
PO Box 41026, Rochester, NY 14604–4126 USA
and of Boydell & Brewer Limited
PO Box 9, Woodbridge, Suffolk IP12 3DF, UK

ISBN: 1–57113–254–6

Library of Congress Cataloging-in-Publication Data

Berg, Henk de, 1963–
 Freud's theory and its use in literary and cultural studies: an introduction
  p. cm. — (Studies in German literature, linguistics, and culture)
 Includes bibliographical references and index.
 ISBN 1–57113–254–6 (hardcover: alk. paper)
  1. Psychoanalysis and literature. 2. Literature, Modern—History and
criticism. 3. Psychoanalysis. I. Title. II. Series.

PN56.P92 B36 2002
809'.93353—dc21

                                                        2002010541

A catalogue record for this title is available from the British Library.

This publication is printed on acid-free paper.
Printed in the United States of America.

Contents

Part Two: Literature and Culture

Preface

THIS BOOK OFFERS AN introduction to Freudian psychoanalysis and its implications for the study of literature and culture. It is written for advanced undergraduate and graduate students, and suitable particularly for literature courses.

The book consists of two parts. Part 1 explains Freud's key ideas, focusing on his theories of repression, of the difference between conscious and unconscious mental processes, and of sexuality; on the role that dreams, free associations, parapraxes (Freudian slips), resistance, and transference play in psychoanalysis; and on the relationship of the ego, superego, and id. The basic assumption underlying this account is that Freud offers not simply a model of the mind, but an analysis of the relation of the individual and society. Part 2 deals with the implications of Freudian psychoanalysis for the study of literature and culture. Although this part also contains a number of theoretical reflections, the emphasis is on the analysis of concrete literary and cultural phenomena. Among the topics discussed are *Hamlet,* Heinrich Heine's "Lore-Ley," fairy tales, Freud's *Totem und Tabu* and its influence on literature, and the German student revolution of the late 1960s.

There are, of course, countless introductions to Freudian psychoanalysis but — surprisingly enough — none that combine an accessible account of Freud's ideas with an introduction to their use in literary and cultural studies. Existing books focus either on Freudian psychoanalysis in general or on psychoanalytic literary and cultural criticism; those that fall into the latter category, moreover, are often fairly abstract and theoretical in nature. None of the existing books are suitable for readers whose primary interest is in psychoanalysis as a tool for literary and cultural criticism but who are relatively unfamiliar with Freud's general theory. This is the audience to which the present study addresses itself.

Throughout, the focus is on classical Freudian psychoanalysis. No attempt is made to introduce the reader to rival psychoanalytic theories or the multifarious ways in which later Freudians have elaborated and revised Freud's ideas. Neither do I discuss the various endeavors to integrate psychoanalysis with structuralist, deconstructionist, feminist, and other critical theories. These shortcomings (if that is the right word) find their justification in the book's intended audience. It is no good trying to run before one can walk. A good grasp of Freud's own ideas is a prerequisite for understanding post-Freudian psychoanalysis. In any case, what Freud has to say is important and interesting enough in itself to warrant a book-length study. In brief, then, this book aims to introduce its readers to the fundamentals of Freudian psychoanalysis; to familiarize them with a number of ways in which Freud's ideas can be used to analyze literary and cultural phenomena; and thus to provide them with the grounding that will enable them to work confidently with more advanced academic material.

Finally, a note on usage. In order to avoid awkward phrases such as *he or she, s/he,* and *him or her,* I have used the masculine pronoun to refer to both sexes.

Acknowledgments

I SHOULD LIKE TO thank my friends and colleagues who commented on the manuscript or helped me in other ways: John Coates, Jaap de Berg, Duncan Large, Moray McGowan, Michael Perraudin, and Karl Wilds.

A Note on Freud's Life and Works

BORN 1856 IN FREIBERG (now Příbor in the Czech Republic). Family settles in Vienna in 1860. Studies medicine at Vienna University, receiving his MD in 1881. Becomes engaged to Martha Bernays and starts working at Vienna General Hospital in 1882. Marries Martha Bernays and sets up private practice in nervous diseases in 1886. Lives and practices in Vienna until Hitler's invasion of Austria in 1938, when he leaves Vienna for London. Dies in London in 1939.

Main Works

1895   *Studien über Hysterie* (Studies on Hysteria; with Josef Breuer).

1899   *Die Traumdeutung* (The Interpretation of Dreams; at the publisher's request, the title page bears the more modern-looking date *1900*).

1901   *Zur Psychopathologie des Alltagslebens* (The Psychopathology of Everyday Life).

1905   *Drei Abhandlungen zur Sexualtheorie* (Three Essays on the Theory of Sexuality) and *Der Witz und seine Beziehung zum Unbewußten* (Jokes and Their Relation to the Unconscious).

1907   *Der Wahn und die Träume in W. Jensens "Gradiva"* (Delusions and Dreams in Jensen's "Gradiva").

1910   *Über Psychoanalyse* (Five Lectures on Psychoanalysis) and *Eine Kindheitserinnerung des Leonardo da Vinci* (Leonardo da Vinci and a Memory of His Childhood).

1913   *Totem und Tabu* (Totem and Taboo).

1914   *Der Moses des Michelangelo* (The Moses of Michelangelo).

1915   *Zeitgemäßes über Krieg und Tod* (Thoughts for the Times on War and Death).

1917   *Vorlesungen zur Einführung in die Psychoanalyse* (Introductory Lectures on Psychoanalysis).

1920   *Jenseits des Lustprinzips* (Beyond the Pleasure Principle).

1921   *Massenpsychologie und Ich-Analyse* (Group Psychology and the Analysis of the Ego).

1923   *Das Ich und das Es* (The Ego and the Id).

1926   *Die Frage der Laienanalyse* (The Question of Lay Analysis).

1927   *Die Zukunft einer Illusion* (The Future of an Illusion).

1930   *Das Unbehagen in der Kultur* (Civilization and Its Discontents).

1933   *Neue Folge der Vorlesungen zur Einführung in die Psychoanalyse* (New Introductory Lectures on Psychoanalysis).

1939   *Der Mann Moses und die monotheistische Religion* (Moses and Monotheism).

Note on Sources and Citations

I HAVE CITED THE STANDARD English translations of Freud's works, but have modified them where I deemed this necessary. Translations from other sources are my own, unless indicated otherwise.

For quotations from Freud, I have used the fifteen-volume *Penguin Freud Library* edited by Angela Richards and Albert Dickson (Harmondsworth: Penguin, 1990–1993), as this edition is more widely available than *The Standard Edition of the Complete Psychological Works of Sigmund Freud*. With the exception of some minor corrections, the translation of the *Penguin Freud Library* is identical to that of the *Standard Edition*. Quotations from Freud's *Five Lectures on Psychoanalysis*, which is not included in the Penguin edition, come from Sigmund Freud, *Two Short Accounts of Psycho-Analysis*, trans. and ed. James Strachey (Harmondsworth: Penguin, 1977).

Part One:
Mind and Society

1: The Birth of Psychoanalysis

PSYCHOANALYSIS HAS PERMEATED the contemporary mind to such an extent that an introduction to its main tenets would seem almost superfluous. *Superego* and *id* have become household names; we are all familiar with Freudian slips; we all know that boys secretly desire their mothers (and girls their fathers), that dreams are wish-fulfillments, and that somehow everything and anything is supposed to be about sex. Is there anything more to it? Well, there is. Besides, the cult status of psychoanalysis has generated a multitude of misconceptions about Freud's ideas. In other words, not only is there more to know than most people know already, but what they think they know is often quite wrong. By way of illustration, let us take a look at a number of popular ideas about Freud and psychoanalysis.

1. Freud discovered the unconscious.

2. The unconscious is the part of the mind we are not conscious of; the conscious is the part we are conscious of.

3. Freud uses the word *subconscious* to highlight the fact that the unconscious is a more hidden, "deeper," region of the mind.

4. Because Freud focuses one-sidedly on the sexual drive, he takes insufficient account of other drives such as aggression.

5. Its subject matter — sexuality in both its normal and abnormal forms — was the biggest obstacle to the scientific and social recognition of psychoanalysis.

6. The superego constitutes what is good in us; the id constitutes what is bad in us.

7. Freud's theory of the mind leaves no room for the analysis of social phenomena.

8. Psychoanalysis is primarily a branch of medicine whose task it is to cure mentally disturbed people.

These statements represent widely held beliefs about Freud and psychoanalysis. *Yet not one of them is correct.* The following two chapters will explain why they are wrong and what it is that Freud does say. In the third chapter, I discuss the revolutionary nature of Freud's ideas. If Freud did not discover the unconscious, then what was new about psychoanalysis? If it was not its frank discussion of the taboo subject of sexuality that made people reject psychoanalysis as immoral, then what did? If psychoanalysis is not simply a branch of medicine that aims to eliminate pathological urges, then what does it seek to achieve? In answering these questions, I shall argue that psychoanalysis is first and foremost a *critical theory of society*. Rather than offering just another model of the mind or of personal development, it provides an analysis of the relationship between individuals and between the individual and society. Nor does Freud try to make people feel better. In a sense, he tries to make them feel worse. He shows people what they are by confronting them with what they do not want to know. Cutting through the layers of self-deception with which society papers over the cracks in its foundations, he questions even our deepest certainties.

Before I can explain this view of psychoanalysis as a form of social critique in more detail, however, we must look at a number of other topics: Freud's study of hysteria; his theories of repression, of the difference between conscious and unconscious mental processes, and of sexuality; the role that dreams, free association, parapraxes (Freudian slips), resistance, and transference play in psychoanalysis; and finally the relationship between the ego, superego, and id and between the id and society. As it was Freud's study of hysteria that led him to develop psychoanalysis, I shall start here.

Hysteria

The history of psychoanalysis begins with a patient called Bertha Pappenheim. She was not Freud's own patient but, from December 1880 until June 1882, had been treated by his older colleague and mentor, Josef Breuer. Together, Breuer and Freud published the case history of Bertha Pappenheim, as well as a number of other case histories, in their *Studien über Hysterie* (Studies on Hysteria, 1895). The ideas triggered by this volume, and especially by the Pappenheim case, set Freud on the track to psychoanalysis.

Bertha Pappenheim or Anna O. (the pseudonym Breuer and Freud used to preserve the patient's anonymity) suffered from what was then called *hysteria*, a catchall term for illnesses without any identifiable cause. Hysterics would exhibit symptoms such as a squint or the inability to move an arm or leg, but a doctor would not be able to find anything wrong with them. Of course there were theories on the cause of hysteria — attributing it to an as yet unexplainable brain disease, for example — but none of them seemed entirely satisfactory. Often hysterics, mostly women, were simply treated as people craving attention. Breuer and Freud took a different view. They came up with a *psychological explanation*. Hysteria had no physical origins, yet neither were hysterics to be looked upon as malingerers. Their physical symptoms were caused by mental processes.

The key to this new explanation lay in Breuer's treatment of Anna O. Breuer had found out that his patient's symptoms disappeared if she could be brought to remember on what occasion they had first appeared and could thereby relieve the mental pressure it had generated. This had not been easy, as she seemed to have forgotten most of these experiences. For example, Anna had been unable to drink; she could quench her thirst only by eating juicy fruit. This situation had persisted for weeks on end. One day, however, Anna unexpectedly "grumbled about her English lady-companion, whom she did not care for, and went on to describe, with every sign of disgust, how she had once gone into that lady's room and how her little dog — horrid creature! — had drunk out of a glass there." Anna, though disgusted by this scene, "had said nothing, as she had wanted to be polite." From then on, she had been unable to drink. But after the patient had related this to Breuer, giving "energetic expression to the anger she had held back," the symptom vanished.[1] Through the same *talking cure* (Anna's own phrase), Breuer had succeeded in eliminating the other symptoms as well. Hence Breuer and Freud concluded that hysterics were suffering from reminiscences; that is, that their symptoms were the result of the continued mental tension produced by traumatic events.

But why does this happen? Why do mental experiences lead to physical symptoms? And why did the symptoms disappear after Anna had told Breuer about their first occurrence? The answer can be found by looking at Anna's difficulty in remembering these occurrences. Anna had suppressed her feelings; she had pushed back her emotions as far back as possible. In the case of the dog drinking from the glass of water, she had swallowed her disgust out of consideration for her lady-companion, and she had done this so successfully that for a long time she was unable to recall the incident. This led Breuer and Freud to the idea that the hysteria had come into being because certain affects, having had their outlet blocked, had to find a new outlet. The strangulated affects, they argued, had undergone a transformation — a transformation into physical symptoms. (A less pathological example of this would be cold sweat when one is frightened, or fiddling with one's hair when one is nervous.) Breuer and Freud called this phenomenon *hysterical conversion*.

Conscious, Preconscious, and Unconscious

Not stopping at the idea of hysterical conversion, Breuer and Freud subjected the process of strangulation to even closer scrutiny. They made two important observations. First, they noted that it was not just any experiences that were suppressed, but wishful impulses — wishful impulses, moreover, that were in conflict with the patients' other wishes and their ethical standards. (Anna O. had wanted to shout at her lady-companion and tell her that allowing her dog to drink from a glass was disgusting, but she had held back so as not to be impolite.) Second, they noted that although these wishful impulses were suppressed — a process for which Freud would later systematically use the term *Verdrängung,* repression — they were still exerting an influence. Had they been expunged, there would have been no need for hysterical conversion; indeed, there would have been nothing left to be converted. So somehow, somewhere, the wishful impulses had to be present, still, in the patient's mind. This convinced Breuer and Freud that there are two different mental processes in the mind, conscious (*bewußt*) processes and unconscious (*unbewußt*) ones. In this way, they arrived at a dualistic model of the mind.

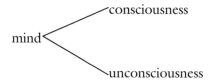

```
              ╱ consciousness
       mind ⟨
              ╲ unconsciousness
```

This idea was of tremendous significance and represented for Freud the first of two major steps towards psychoanalysis. (The second, as we shall see in a moment, was the discovery of the decisive part that sexuality plays in hysteria, and indeed in life generally; an idea that Breuer was not prepared to accept.) Despite, or perhaps because of, the significance of this model of the mind, there are many myths surrounding it. I wish to address four of them.

First of all, the dualistic model of the mind was so important because it differed radically from most other approaches at the time, not because it was totally new. Breuer and Freud helped to give the scientific study of the mind a new direction, but they did not discover the unconscious. Others, including philosophers such as Arthur Schopenhauer (1788–1860) and Friedrich Nietzsche (1844–1900), had already developed similar ideas. Still, the majority of scholars studying mental processes towards the end of the nineteenth century, mostly biologists and neurologists, saw the human mind in purely physical terms. To them, the mind was the brain, an organ like any other; more complicated perhaps, but not essentially different. Any speculation about nonphysical entities was just that: idle speculation, unscientific eyewash. It was Breuer's and Freud's achievement to regain the "unscientific" concept of the unconscious, to put it at the center of their theory of the mind, and to demonstrate that it possesses empirical validity.

Second, the correct word is *unconscious,* not *subconscious.* Expressions such as "the subconscious mind" or "I did it subconsciously" are un-Freudian. This is not just a matter of terminology, but of theory. The word *subconscious* suggests a deeper, lower region of the mind, just as *subcutaneous* means "below the skin surface." But to conceive of the unconscious in spatial terms is a mistake, albeit an understandable one (in explaining the unconscious Freud frequently uses spatial metaphors). Like the conscious, the unconscious is not a place but a process, always active, always in motion, always exerting its influence. Therefore, to think of the unconscious as a kind of cellar where we stack away our unwanted urges and memories is to overlook its most fundamental feature, dynamism. Our unconscious is a force that is always operative, not some Pandora's box, effective only when its contents are brought to the light of day. At any given moment, the human mind is an interplay of consciousness and unconsciousness.[2]

Third, the unconscious is not equivalent to everything we are not conscious of. There are many things that most of the time we are not conscious of: our telephone number, the wonderful holiday we had last year, the intention to see our parents more often, the decision to lose weight, and so on. All these things that we are not constantly aware of but which we can call to mind any time are, in Freud's terminology, *vorbewußt*, preconscious. Unconscious, by contrast, are those things that we are not aware of and which we cannot recall even when we try. To be more precise, the unconscious comprises what we have *repressed*, either recently or a long time ago. Of course, the same mental content, let us say a holiday memory, can be both preconscious and unconscious (though obviously not at the same time). If simply not thought of, it is preconscious; if repressed, it is unconscious. Moreover, the same mental content can alternate between consciousness and unconsciousness. Something awful happens and is repressed; coming back, it is repressed again, and so on.

Fourth, the dualistic model (conscious/unconscious) is not Freud's final word on the workings of the mind. In fact, during his long and highly productive life Freud developed *several* theories of the mind, and one of the problems in reading Freud is that the relationship between these various theories is not always clear. We shall look at the most important other theory, the tripartite model (ego/superego/id), in chapter 3.

What are the implications of the model of the mind as an aggregate of conscious and unconscious processes? What does it mean for the problem of hysteria? It means, Breuer and Freud argued, that hysterics such as Anna O. suffer from *unsuccessful repression*. Hysterics are people who have failed in their attempts to repress certain wishful impulses and are therefore faced with hysterical conversion. Their wishful impulses have not been pushed out of consciousness successfully but have slipped back in again, albeit it in a different form; to wit, as the physical symptoms of hysteria. So the problem is not the existence of unconscious processes as such. *Every* person's mind consists of both conscious and unconscious processes. Neither is the attempt at repression the problem. *Everyone* is continually repressing things. The problem is the failure to repress successfully, and the solution is to help the patient to abandon his vain attempts at repression and to confront his wishful impulses. Of course, this does not necessarily amount to urging the patient to act out those impulses. There are other ways of dealing with one's wishes: rejecting them consciously, for instance, or trying to find suitable alternatives.

In this way, Breuer and Freud managed to explain hysteria. Breuer was satisfied with this. Freud, however, was not. He wanted to know exactly what kind of wishes are repressed. After all, seeing an animal drink from a glass normally used by a human being may be disgusting, but it is hardly sufficient to explain a phobia for liquid. The real cause of hysteria, Freud thought, must lie deeper.[3]

Sexuality

Through his theoretical and therapeutic work, Freud discovered that what is repressed is always, in some way or another, related to *sexuality*. What is repressed is not simply every affect, but sexual wishes or at least affects that are derived from or associated with sexual wishes. This was the decisive step towards psychoanalysis, a step that Freud had to take on his own, for here Breuer was not prepared to follow.[4]

When referring to these sexual wishes, Freud usually uses the word *Triebe*. This is often translated as "instincts," but "drives" is more adequate. Instincts are relevant only at certain times, not at others (as with a bird's instinct to build a nest or migrate to a warmer climate), whereas our *Triebe* are always driving us, always influencing us, always pushing for satisfaction, always trying to get the upper hand. That is why I said in the previous section that the unconscious is not a place, but a process. Moreover, drives can be suppressed and, as we shall see throughout this book, redirected or even changed into their opposites: love can be transformed into hatred, desire into revulsion. Instincts, by contrast, are fixed and immutable.

Sexual drives do not only occur in adult life but also in childhood. As a matter of fact, they are there from birth onwards. The sex-drive, Freud says, does not enter "into children at the age of puberty in the way in which, in the Gospel, the devil entered into the swine," but "comes into the world with them."[5] Our whole life is thus a constant interplay of unconscious sexual drives and conscious decisions. But although our whole life is an interplay of unconsciousness and consciousness, it is our childhood that sets the stage for what we become. It is the interplay of unconsciousness and consciousness in childhood that determines what kind of adult we become, including how vulnerable we are going to be to potentially traumatic experiences (as with Anna O. and the glass of water).

The notions of infantile sexuality and, perhaps even more so, of the omnipresence of the sex-drive in our lives are among the most contested of Freud's many controversial positions. Children, it is objected, do not have sexual wishes; they are looking for love, attention, sympathy, understanding, not sex. Or, granted that sexuality plays an important role in our lives, are not other drives such as aggression just as important? However, these and similar objections miss the point of what Freud is saying. Let me quote him at some length. The child's sex-drive

> serves for the acquisition of different kinds of pleasurable feeling, which, basing ourselves on analogies and connections, we bring together under the idea of sexual pleasure. The chief source of infantile sexual pleasure is the appropriate excitation of certain parts of the body that are especially susceptible to stimulus; apart from the genitals, these are the oral, anal, and urethral orifices, as well as the skin and other sensory surfaces. Since at this first phase of infantile sexual life satisfaction is obtained from the child's own body and extraneous objects are disregarded, we term this phase (from a word coined by Havelock Ellis) that of *auto-erotism*. We call the parts of the body that are important in the acquisition of sexual pleasure "erotogenic zones." Thumb-sucking (or sensual sucking) in the youngest infants is a good example of this auto-erotic satisfaction from an erotogenic zone. . . . Another sexual satisfaction at this period of life is the masturbatory excitation of the genitals. . . . Alongside these and other auto-erotic activities, we find in children at a very early age manifestations of those components of sexual pleasure (or, as we like to say, of libido) which presuppose the taking of an extraneous person as an object. These drives occur in pairs of opposites, active and passive. I may mention as the most important representatives of this group the desire to cause pain (sadism) with its passive counterpart (masochism) and voyeurism and exhibitionism. . . . [And then there are also] the coprophilic impulses of childhood; that is to say, the desires attaching to the excreta. . . . But here you will perhaps protest that all this is not sexuality. I use the word in a far wider sense than that in which you have been accustomed to understand it.[6]

When Freud uses the terms *sexuality* and *sexual*, then, he does not simply refer to genital sexuality or to other forms of what is usually considered to be sexuality. *He uses these terms in a much wider sense to denote any kind of sensual pleasure*, a sense which includes things like having sex or being sexually aroused, but extends beyond them. For Freud, any pleasurable excitation of the senses is sexual: the feeling a baby experiences when sucking at its mother's breast or at the bottle, a child's happiness when sucking its thumb, the satisfaction some of us derive from shouting at an arrogant but incompetent shop assistant, the good feeling we can get from punching a particularly nasty person (or from thinking about this), and so on. Even going to the toilet can be sexual. All of us have at times experienced the pleasurable feeling when, after a long walk or a long meeting, we can finally relieve ourselves; a feeling which sometimes might even resemble an orgasm.

As I have already noted, a key characteristic of sexuality in the wider sense is that it is there from birth onwards. That is why Freud describes babies and small children as being *polymorphously perverse*. They are perverts because they unashamedly derive pleasure from such things as thumb-sucking and defecation — something most adults would be too embarrassed to do (or at least too embarrassed to admit to) in public. This perversion is termed polymorphous ("having many forms") because children derive pleasure from all or at least many of these things, and not just, as with most adult perverts, from one or a few of them. In this sense, all babies and small children are *sex-monsters,* focused on satisfying all their sensual urges, without shame and without regard for the feelings of others. Only as they grow up do they learn to be ashamed of deriving pleasure from defecation, masturbation, and the like, and to harmonize the satisfaction of their urges with the needs and interests of others.

But why does Freud call all these activities sexual? Why does he not simply say "sensual pleasure" or "the search for happiness"? Freud argues that if we did not consider the pleasure we derive from something like defecation as sexual, then it would be impossible to explain sexual deviations such as coprophilia or indeed to explain the sexual orientation of adults generally. Only if we view things such as sucking at the mother's breast and defecating not merely as the consumption and excretion of food, but also as sexual activities, will we be able to explain a person's sexual development. Why this is so, and what forms this development can take — these are questions to which we must now turn.

From Polymorphous Perversity to Adult Sexuality

All babies and small children are polymorphously perverse. They derive sensual pleasure from a variety of body zones, and they do so without shame or guilt. However, not all these ways of obtaining sensual (in Freud's terminology, sexual) satisfaction are approved of by society. Some are, understandably, seen as a nuisance or a danger. Children cannot be allowed to relieve themselves whenever and wherever they want, and they certainly cannot be allowed to satisfy their aggressive urges indiscriminately. Other ways to sensual satisfaction are frowned upon for less obvious reasons. Masturbation, for example, was condemned by virtually everyone in the late nineteenth and early twentieth centuries (including Freud) and even today is still pretty much taboo. In addition, individual parents, teachers, and other educators have *personal* likes and dislikes that lead them to approve or disapprove of a child's actions. The society and the period in which a child grows up, his immediate social environment (parents, teachers, and so on), and of course a number of contingent circumstances such as the possible death of a parent or, less dramatically, a move to a different city — all these factors taken together determine the course of the child's development into sexual adulthood.

Before I explain this in more concrete terms, however, I should mention a problem with Freud's approach: it neglects biological factors. By this I do not mean that Freud *rejects* the idea that our biological make-up affects our personal development. He knew about hereditary diseases, and in several passages he refers to the possible influence of biological and biochemical factors on mental processes. But he does not have much to say about this link, and his whole theory is based on psychological rather than biological considerations. Many critics see this as a serious shortcoming of Freud's theory. Given the discoveries in genetics over the last few decades it is not hard to understand their position. Yet only time can tell whether they are right. As long as there are no convincing theories of the relationship between genetic make-up and

personality, psychology is all we are left with. Moreover, although ge-
neticists may sooner or later provide explanations for certain *parts* of our
personality, it seems unlikely that the medical and biological sciences will
ever completely replace the psychological study of the mind — the study
of the way our personality develops and achieves unity as a result of
mental processes that take shape in the interaction with a specific social
environment.

Let us now examine the various ways in which, according to Freud,
children grow into sexual adulthood. The first is what might be called
normal sexual development. In this context, the word *normal* is not used
in an evaluative sense. It simply means "in accordance with what most
people happen to think or do." Normal sexual development leads to
heterosexuality and usually, in Freud's time as in ours, to a marriage with
children. In order to arrive at this sexual orientation, a number of the
child's original drives need to be repressed; its unabashed pleasure in
defecating, for instance, needs to be curbed by toilet-training. Other
sexual drives such as voyeurism may be repressed, or satisfied as part of
one's sex-life.

Repressing and acting out alone are not sufficient for a normal sexual
development. Many drives are too strong simply to be repressed, and
acting them out often proves impossible (because we are too ashamed,
because our partner is not willing to participate, or because law or morality forbids it). These drives are then satisfied through fantasies and a
variety of *cultural pursuits* such as reading or writing literary texts. For
these culturally oriented forms of satisfaction, Freud uses a special word:
Sublimierung, sublimation, the diversion of sexual energy into a culturally higher activity. (The Latin verb *sublimare* means "raise," "place in
an elevated position.") Drawing an analogy with hysterical conversion —
the transformation of wishful impulses into the symptoms of hysteria —
one could speak of *cultural conversion,* the transformation of wishful
impulses into "symptoms" of culture such as literature and art. With a
more drastic analogy, to masturbation, one could speak of "read-
ing/writing oneself off," although people are rarely aware that this is
what they are doing. Reading and writing are forms of unconscious
mental masturbation.

The theory of sublimation has important implications for the study
of literature, art, and indeed culture generally. It implies that cultural

products must be seen as ways in which people deal with their sexual drives; even though, again, they are not conscious of the fact that this is what they are doing. A psychoanalytic interpretation of literary texts and of the reactions to these texts can therefore tell us a good deal about people's unconscious wishes, about how they have or have not been able to fulfill these wishes, about their upbringing, and about their interaction with their social environment. In other words, it can tell us a good deal not just about the texts themselves, but also about their authors and readers. I shall illustrate this in detail in part 2. Here I only wish to point out that although sublimation sounds very "arty" and is often interpreted as such, it does not have to be. Cultural conversion takes place in many different ways. To borrow two examples from Calvin Hall, "a lawyer may get a great deal of oral gratification from arguing a case before a jury, a surgeon may find an outlet for his aggressive urges by operating upon patients."[7] Moreover, the process is not restricted to man's more elevated cultural achievements. Pornography, too, is a form of sublimation, and so is looking at the models in *Playboy*.

Even the writing and reading of academic texts on Freud can fulfill a sublimatory function. This does not mean that they are nothing more than forms of sublimation. One of the things Freud stresses again and again is that most phenomena are *überdeterminiert,* overdetermined; in other words, that there is more than one reason for them. These reasons can be of a sexual nature, but they do not have to be. For example, one can watch David Lynch's or Roman Polanski's films because they are erotic, but at the same time because watching such films makes one look intellectual or because they are the topic of a university course one is taking. Often, the various reasons are intertwined in a highly complex way. From a logical point of view they can even be contradictory: doing the dishes for your girlfriend in order to help her but also, unconsciously, in order to punish her by making her feel guilty.

We now move on to the second way into adulthood, the way to an abnormal sexuality, to perversion. As with the word *normal,* the words *abnormal* and *perversion* are not meant in an evaluative sense. In Freud's work they simply mean "what most people happen to find abnormal or perverted." As a person, Freud shared these assessments or prejudices in some cases; in others he was considerably more tolerant than the majority of his contemporaries. Someone develops an abnormal sexuality if he remains stuck in a stage others grow out of. This, according to Freud, is the case with bisexuality. We are all born bisexual, he says, but most of us develop a preference for the opposite sex. There is also the possibility that components of the child's polymorphous perversity, instead of being integrated into a normal sex-life, become autonomous. People then develop into voyeurs, exhibitionists, or sadists.

Finally, there is the third way into adulthood — a less happy way than the two others. Not all people manage to deal with their original drives successfully. Normal people do so by repressing them, perverts by acting them out (as long as they do not break the law, there is no problem). There are people, however, who do not succeed in repressing their drives but are at the same time incapable of acting them out without feeling guilty. They are the ones who have repressed unsuccessfully: the unhappy homosexual, the bisexual who keeps trying to push back this other part of himself, and so on. Sometimes, the half-repressed drives find other outlets; the sexual tension is then converted into hysterical or neurotic symptoms.

The differences among these three ways into adulthood are not as clear-cut as the above may seem to suggest. For example, no clear demarcation exists between people who "like it rough" on the one hand, and sadists and masochists on the other. There is, however, a much more fundamental sense in which the classification above is misleading. Here, we touch upon one of the essential insights of Freudian psychoanalysis, the normality of perversion.

The Normality of Perversion

Why is the classification I have just outlined fundamentally misleading? The answer is to be found in the nature of the unconscious. The unconscious, I said, is not a kind of Pandora's box, inactive when closed, but a process. It is always active, always struggling for expression. Repression therefore needs to be a constant process too. But however hard we repress the drives of the unconscious, we can never make them go away. The unconscious always keeps pushing back. Hence, all the drives that constitute the child's polymorphous perversity are to be found in adults too: in perverts, in neurotics, in hysterics, *and in normal people*. Normal people are simply people who have repressed their drives to a greater extent than other people but, again, *repressed does not mean eliminated.* The unconscious is always on the lookout for an outlet, in all of us.

One only needs to look at the atrocious crimes committed in wartime to understand what Freud is getting at. Take rape as an example. I am convinced that none of my male readers has ever seriously considered raping a woman. (If anyone has, he ought to be locked up). Yet rape, including the sexual excitement that is the condition for carrying it out, is one of the most frequent crimes in wartime. No society, no individual is ever safe from what Freud calls *die Wiederkehr des Verdrängten,* the return of the repressed. When the incentives for repression fall away, our darkest desires reappear. As Freud put it when commenting on the disillusionment that so many people felt at what apparently civilized nations were doing to each other in the First World War:

> In reality our fellow-citizens have not sunk so low as we feared, because they had never risen so high as we believed.[8]

It is not only wars and other exceptional situations that reveal the monster within us. It suffices, Freud says, to look at the dreams that people, even perfectly ordinary people, dream. The psychoanalytic interpretation of dreams shows "that whenever we go to sleep we throw off our hard-won morality like a garment, and put it on again next morning."[9] (I shall examine Freud's theory of dreams in more detail in chapter 2.) There is, then, only a quantitative, not a qualitative difference between *us* (normal people) and *them* (perverts). This is one of the key insights of Freudian psychoanalysis: that deep down *all* of us are monsters, that man's badness can never be eradicated, and that the repressed can return at any time.

It would be a fundamental mistake, however, to conclude from this that all people are equally bad or that it is irrelevant how perverted one is. The distinction between normal people (that is, potential perverts) and sadists and other abnormal people (that is, actual perverts) may be only quantitative, but that does not make the distinction less important. There is, after all, quite a difference between consciously or unconsciously *thinking* about bashing someone's head in and actually *doing* it. In other words, what Freud questions is the absolute nature of the distinction, not the distinction itself.

Neither does Freud's theory imply that all our attempts to act morally are pointless. On the contrary, precisely because we have these urges within us, it is essential that we try to be as moral as we realistically can. Also, there is no reason to assume that man is not made to be moral, that culture is essentially artificial, and that we can only really be ourselves if we cut ourselves loose from the demands society places upon us. To assume this would be to fall victim to the genetic fallacy, the mistaken idea that because something comes first temporally, it is somehow primary or more valuable. We may be born polymorphous perverts, focused on the satisfaction of our sensual urges, but we are also social beings, unable to live without the help, love, and understanding of other social beings. Therefore, it is only when we find a balance between our urges and the requirements of the social world around us that we can be at ease with ourselves.

Notes

[1] Josef Breuer and Sigmund Freud, *Studies on Hysteria,* trans. James Strachey, ed. James Strachey and Angela Richards, vol. 3 of *The Penguin Freud Library,* ed. Angela Richards and Albert Dickson (Harmondsworth: Penguin, 1991), 88.

[2] This explanation of the theoretical inadequacy of the phrase *subconscious* is perhaps more my own than Freud's. Freud himself never discussed the reason, or reasons, for his aversion to the phrase in any detail. It appears he objected to it most of all because it could be interpreted as denoting merely an undeveloped form of consciousness. An additional reason may have been that the phrase was used by Pierre Janet (1859–1947), a French competitor of Freud's. Freud did actually use *subconscious* a few times in the 1890s, but quickly abandoned it. Yet even *Studien über Hysterie,* in which the word *is* on occasion used, warns against its misleading spatial connotations: "It is only too easy to fall into a habit of thought which assumes that every substantive [i.e., noun] has a substance behind it and which comes to regard 'consciousness' as a thing, an object; and when we have become accustomed to make use metaphorically of spatial relations, as in the term 'subconsciousness,' we find as time goes on that we have actually formed an image which has lost its metaphorical nature and which we treat all too easily as if it were real. Our mythology is then complete. All our thinking tends to be accompanied and aided by spatial images, and we talk in spatial metaphors. Thus when we speak of ideas which are found in the region of clear consciousness and of unconscious ones which never enter the full light of self-consciousness, we almost inevitably form pictures of a tree with its trunk in daylight and its roots in darkness, or of a building with its dark underground cellars. If,

however, we constantly bear in mind that all such spatial relations are metaphorical and do not allow ourselves to be seduced into allocating to them specific locations in the brain, we may nevertheless speak of a consciousness and a subconsciousness. But only on this condition" (Breuer and Freud, *Studies on Hysteria,* 306–7; translation modified).

[3] For Anna O., this insight came too late. Although in *Studien über Hysterie* Breuer suggests otherwise, her symptoms recurred almost immediately after he had concluded his treatment of her. Over the next few years, she spent a considerable amount of time in sanatoriums. She later became a well-known social worker, but it is not clear whether she ever recovered completely. In fact, the circumstances surrounding Breuer's failed treatment are still partly shrouded in mystery. This does not, of course, diminish the historical significance of the Anna O. case, which lies in the crucial part it played in the development of Freud's thinking.

[4] There was another difference between Freud and Breuer that is worth mentioning. Breuer had treated Anna O. by applying *hypnosis* in order to put her into a state conducive to psychiatric treatment and facilitate the retrieval of her suppressed emotions. Freud, by contrast, grew dissatisfied with this method. Working with the other patients that were to become the subject of *Studien über Hysterie,* he discovered that only a tiny minority of his patients were capable of being hypnotized. More importantly, it became evident that hypnosis, while rendering some mental processes accessible, obscured the precise nature of a patient's repressions. Freud therefore gradually abandoned hypnosis, replacing it first with the so-called *pressure-technique* (putting his hand on the patient's forehead and urging him on by pressing each time the flow of information seemed to dry up) and eventually with genuinely *psychoanalytic techniques* such as free association. These will be examined in chapter 2.

[5] Sigmund Freud, *Five Lectures on Psychoanalysis,* in *Two Short Accounts of Psycho-Analysis,* trans. and ed. James Strachey (Harmondsworth: Penguin, 1977), 71.

[6] Freud, *Five Lectures on Psychoanalysis,* 73–76; translation modified.

[7] Calvin S. Hall, *A Primer of Freudian Psychology* (New York: Mentor/New American Library, 1954), 83.

[8] Sigmund Freud, *Civilisation, Society and Religion,* trans. James Strachey, vol. 12 of *The Penguin Freud Library,* ed. Albert Dickson (Harmondsworth: Penguin, 1991), 72.

[9] Freud, *Civilisation, Society and Religion,* 73.

2: How to Gain Access to the Unconscious

NOT EVERYONE MANAGES TO FIND a balance between inner urges and social demands. Sometimes people fail to repress the things they unconsciously wish to repress, and the strangulated affects are converted into physical symptoms. Or, alternatively, they repress their drives to the extent of losing touch with this part of themselves and feel strangely empty as a result. In some cases, the reasons for the imbalance can be found in the nature of the social demands; one only needs to think of the uncompromising expectations of moral propriety placed on middle-class women in Freud's Vienna or Victorian England. In other cases, the imbalance between inner urges and social demands is rooted in individual circumstances.

Regardless of whether the roots are of a more social or a more individual nature, the question that arises is the same: what can be done about the imbalance? How can a more stable state of mind be achieved? The obvious solution is to change the social or personal conditions. Here, however, we run into a serious difficulty. For what are these social and personal conditions that need changing? What precisely is it that someone with hysterical symptoms or someone who feels empty is suffering from? This seems impossible to tell because the processes we are dealing with are unconscious. The urges have been pushed out of consciousness and have therefore become unconscious. The process of repression itself is something one is not aware of either, as it is impossible consciously to repress something. One cannot get something out of one's head by constantly telling oneself: I must get this out of my head.[1] This makes identifying the roots of a person's problems extremely difficult.

So what can be done? How can unconscious processes be made conscious? Long and intense conversations might help, with the psychoanalyst trying to penetrate the patient's mind as deeply as possible. But this alone will seldom, if ever, be sufficient. For the patient has repressed things precisely in order *not* to know them anymore. Hence, the better the psychoanalyst does, the less the patient (unconsciously) will want to cooperate. As Freud puts it, the patient will start putting up an unconscious *Widerstand,* resistance, to the psychoanalyst's attempts to help him. Therefore, the psychoanalyst has to find a way to gather information about his patient's mental processes without asking him directly. Freud developed four such techniques: the interpretation of dreams; the interpretation of slips of the tongue and other "Freudian slips"; the interpretation of free associations; and the interpretation of resistance and transference.

The Interpretation of Dreams I

According to Freud's *Die Traumdeutung* (The Interpretation of Dreams, issued in 1899 with the title page postdated to 1900), all dreams are meaningful. This in itself is not a new idea. Many people have believed that dreams contain open or coded messages. What *is* new is Freud's understanding of the kind of messages that can be found in dreams, and his explanation of how these messages are produced.

Every dream, Freud says, contains both a manifest dream-content (*ein manifester Trauminhalt*) and a latent dream-thought (*ein latenter Traumgedanke*).

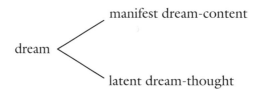

The manifest dream-content is the dream as we remember it after we have woken up. The latent dream-thought is what we might call the dream's hidden message. This is as a rule an unconscious wish. In order to understand why this should be so and why this wish is not openly expressed in the dream, we need to look into the mechanism controlling our dreams.

Human beings constantly repress many wishes. They do so because of what other people say (as with children whose parents tell them to "behave" and "control themselves") or because they find their wishes morally reprehensible (as with Anna O., who did not want to hurt her lady-companion's feelings) or because they cannot put up with the inability to act out their wishes (as with many women in Victorian England). Wishes, in other words, get repressed because they contravene social norms and values that the individual has accepted, or has been forced to accept, as his own. Thus, repression occurs because there is a clash between the individual's wishes and his social conscience. The social conscience wins out, and the wishes are pushed out of consciousness and keep being pushed out of consciousness.

Our social conscience is less powerful while we are sleeping. It is not engaged in any interaction with the outside world and is therefore less vigilant. As a result, the repression is weaker and our unconscious wishes stand a much better chance of becoming conscious. This is what happens in the dream. *In the dream, our unconscious wishes become conscious.* They do so, however, *in a distorted form.* For although our social conscience is weaker while we are sleeping, it is not completely inactive. Therefore, even in our sleep our wishes still count as morally reprehensible. So what happens is that they do manage to become conscious, but in a modified form, a form more acceptable to our social conscience. To put it simply, they get censored. Instead of dreaming what we really want (say, bashing the boss's head in), we dream about something less immoral (having a heated argument with him or insulting him). In Freud's own succinct formulation:

a dream is a (disguised) fulfilment of a (suppressed or repressed) wish.[2]

This theory of dreams raises several questions. Before we look at them, though, let us examine the censorship process in more detail. How does this process work? How does the dream transform morally reprehensible wishes into something more acceptable? What, in other words, are the mechanisms underlying what Freud calls *Traumarbeit,* the dream-work? Freud identifies five mechanisms: *Symbolisierung,* or symbolization; *Dramatisierung,* or dramatization; *Verschiebung,* or displacement; *Verdichtung,* or condensation; and *sekundäre Bearbeitung,* or secondary revision. Let us take them in succession.

Symbolization is the most famous, or perhaps one should say infamous, of them all. Through symbolization, things, persons, activities — in short, any object of mental processes — are turned into symbols that stand for these things, persons, and activities. Taking the crudest of examples, the penis may be symbolized by pointed objects such as pens and umbrellas; the vagina by receptacles such as boxes and pots. This area of psychoanalysis, perhaps more than any other, has caught the public imagination, becoming an endless source of everyday amateur psychologizing and embarrassing "knob jokes." Even the advertising industry has seized upon these Freudian symbols.

Because this part of psychoanalytic theory has become so popular, it is important to stress that the relation between the symbol and what it stands for is not predetermined. The meaning of a dream image — a pen, an umbrella, whatever it may be — can never be known in advance, but only in relation to the dream as a whole and the dreamer's personal history. For one dreamer, a gun may be related to sexual intercourse, for another to aggression, for a third to something else again. Moreover, pens, umbrellas, boxes, and the like do not have to act as symbols. As Freud is supposed to have said (although there is no evidence that he did say it): sometimes a cigar is just a cigar. That is why all "Dream Symbols from A to Z" type of books are nothing but eyewash (and why Freud himself is on pretty thin ice when, in the later editions of his own book on dreams and against the thrust of his own theory, he keeps adding information on what particular dream symbols "usually" mean).[3]

Pens can stand for the penis because they have a similar shape. But symbolization does not have to be based on similarity. Anything that, in the dreamer's mind, is associated with *x* can act as a symbol of *x*. A painting can symbolize the person who painted it, a hat can symbolize the person who wears it, sweat can symbolize hard work, a railway station can symbolize death. In linguistic terms, the relationship between the symbol and what it stands for can be both of a metaphorical nature (that is, based on similarity) and of a metonymical nature (that is, based not on similarity but on any other type of association: *pars pro toto* [a part for the whole], *totum pro parte* [the whole for a part], contiguity, and so on).

The second mechanism underlying the dream-work is *dramatization*, the translation of wishes, or any mental content related to them, into an image or a sequence of images. Here are two examples from Freud.

A lady had the following dream: *A servant girl was standing on a ladder as if she were cleaning a window, and had a chimpanzee with her and a gorilla-cat* (the dreamer afterwards corrected this to *an angora cat*). *She hurled the animals at the dreamer; the chimpanzee cuddled up to her, which was very disgusting.* — This dream achieved its purpose by an extremely simple device: it took a figure of speech literally and gave an exact representation of its wording. "Monkey" and animals' names in general are used as invectives; and the situation in the dream meant neither more nor less than "hurling invectives."[4]

The dream-work adopted a slightly different method in the following instance. The dream referred to an excursion to the Hilmteich [a stretch of water on the outskirts of the town] near Graz. *The weather outside was fearful. There was a wretched hotel, water was dripping from the walls of the room, the bed-clothes were damp.* (The latter part of the dream was reported less directly than I have given it.) The meaning of the dream was "superfluous" [*überflüssig*]. This abstract idea, which was present in the dream-thoughts, was in the first instance given a somewhat forced twist and put into some such form as "overflowing," "flowing over" or "fluid" — after which it was represented in a number of similar pictures: water outside, water on the walls inside, water in the dampness of the bed-clothes — everything flowing or "overflowing" [*"über"flüssig*].[5]

The third mechanism involves the *displacement* of an idea concerning one person onto another. For example, you unconsciously want to sleep with your mother, but you dream about sleeping with one of her friends. Like symbolization, displacement has become one of the clichés of psychoanalysis and a source of ridicule and parody. Take only the following scene from Billy Wilder's well-known 1974 film *The Front Page,* in which quintessential Hollywood psychoanalyst Dr. Eggelhofer (bow-tie, spectacles, heavy German accent) questions someone accused of murdering a policeman.

Dr. Eggelhofer: Tell me about your father.

Earl Williams: My father was a train conductor.

Dr. Eggelhofer: Ah! So your father wore a uniform, just like ze policeman. Zat is very significant. Now tell me about your youth.

Earl Williams: I had a perfectly ordinary youth.

Dr. Eggelhofer: So you wanted to kill your father and sleep
with your mother.
Earl Williams: (turning to the sheriff) If he starts talking filth,
I'm out of here!

It is clear what Eggelhofer is implying: Earl Williams unconsciously
wanted to kill his father and displaced this death-wish onto the policeman, whom he then killed.

Billy Wilder's parody is not only evidence of the classic status of the
displacement mechanism (and, of course, of the Oedipus complex, to
which I shall turn in part 2). It also illustrates that according to psychoanalysis displacement may occur not only in dreams, but in real life as
well. In everyday life, too, people unconsciously displace feelings they
have for one person onto another. If we step back from Wilder's parody
and look at our own lives, it is not hard to find examples. We frequently
take out on our partners the anger we feel towards our friends. Or we
ascribe our own dislike of someone, not to ourselves, but to the person
we dislike: "I do not have a problem with him. It is he who hates *me*."
Guilty feelings, too, often lead to displacement: "We did not behave
irresponsibly towards our child. It is the baby-sitter who is to blame."

Condensation takes place when the dream blends different ideas. This
process occurs together with symbolization or dramatization: different
ideas are blended into one symbol or image. In the section on symbolization above, we saw that one symbol or image can have different
meanings. A pen sometimes symbolizes the penis, sometimes the person
who owns the pen, sometimes someone who is particularly fond of pens,
sometimes hard work, sometimes the ambition to become a writer, and
so on. Now in the case of condensation the symbol or image means
several things *at the same time*. For example, when a woman dreams
about buying a hat, this can signify that she wants her sister to die (hat
= mourning hat) and her husband to make love to her (hat = penis).

The process of condensation may even combine contradictory ideas.
Thus, buying a hat can symbolize that one has both a death-wish and a
sex-wish towards someone. The simultaneous existence of contradictory
ideas is not as strange as it may seem. I already mentioned the example
of the man who does the dishes for his girlfriend because he wants to
help her *and* because (unconsciously) he wants to make her feel guilty.

We shall encounter other examples later on. Indeed, we shall see that according to psychoanalysis virtually all feelings are mixed with other, often quite different feelings.

The final dream-work mechanism is *sekundäre Bearbeitung,* secondary revision. (The older, somewhat misleading translation is *secondary elaboration.*) Secondary revision links up individual symbols and images by establishing causal and chronological links between them. Freud's explanation of this mechanism is not particularly clear, but the idea seems to run as follows. In the dream, our deepest desires manage to manifest themselves. But they do so in a civilized disguise. The dream-work subjects them to processes of symbolization, dramatization, displacement, and condensation to make them more acceptable to our social conscience. One could describe these processes, with a term Freud does not use himself, as forms of *primary revision.* The result of this transformation are individual symbols and images, which are combined into a story by another process of transformation acting "in the manner which the poet maliciously ascribes to philosophers: it fills up the gaps in the dream-structure with shreds and patches."[6] This is the *secondary revision;* an infelicitous phrase, as the insertion of narrative putty is supposed to take place, not after, but at the same time as the primary revision. Freud seems to assume that this process, too, is a form of censorship, because in his view the story that emerges is even further removed from our original wishes than are the symbols and images. It is not clear, however, whether this is always the case. In some editions of *Die Traumdeutung,* Freud does not classify secondary revision as a dream-work mechanism proper; that is, not as a form of censorship. What is more, Freud at times talks about the story as a whole, not just the individual symbols and images, as expressing our repressed wishes. This lack of theoretical clarity makes this concept difficult to work with.

The Interpretation of Dreams II:
Some Problems

Freud describes the interpretation of dreams as "*the royal road to a knowledge of the unconscious activities of the mind.*"[7] This seems rather optimistic. In fact, the psychoanalytic theory of dreams is not without its difficulties. To begin with, it is hard to apply. Or perhaps it would be better to say that it is almost too easy to apply. I have already pointed out the elastic nature of the concept of secondary revision. But the other dream-work mechanisms, too, leave the psychoanalyst a substantial amount of interpretive freedom. Is a pen just a pen, or does it have symbolic meaning? If so, what does it stand for — a penis, a thin man, an office job, someone called Penn, or something else again? Or does it stand for several of these things simultaneously (condensation)? Similar questions can be asked with respect to dramatization. Add to this the possibility of displacement, and it becomes clear that the psychoanalytic interpretation of dreams is by no means the safe road to the unconscious Freud would have us believe.

Given this interpretive latitude, it is not surprising that many critics have rejected Freudian dream-analysis as hopelessly subjective and therefore unworkable. Yet in defense of Freud it should be pointed out that interpretation is seldom a straightforward process. Certainly the interpretation of historical events and of cultural products such as literary texts never is, and it would be surprising if the interpretation of dreams were any different. The problem, then, resides not so much in the interpretive latitude as such. The problem — or the challenge — facing Freudian dream-analysis is that its results should be plausible. Such plausibility can only be achieved, first, if the interpretation of dreams is combined with other forms of psychoanalytic access to the unconscious (with the interpretation of Freudian slips, free associations, resistance, and transference) and, second, if the dreamer's personal history is taken into account. In this way, interpretive assumptions relating to the dreamer's dreams can be supported, corrected, or rejected by information gained through interpretive assumptions relating to his personal history, Freudian slips, free associations, and so on.

It would therefore be unfair to say that the psychoanalytic interpretation of dreams amounts to no more than subjective guesswork or that the psychoanalyst can make the dream mean anything he wants it to mean. There is a criterion, if not of truth, then at least of plausibility. This criterion is the compatibility of the interpretive results with other information about the dreamer's consciousness and unconsciousness that the psychoanalyst possesses. All this does mean, however, that the interpretation of dreams cannot convincingly be seen as "the securest foundation of psycho-analysis,"[8] as Freud himself would have it. It is not a privileged way into the unconscious, but makes sense only when combined with other, equally valid, psychoanalytic techniques.

There is another possible objection to Freudian dream-analysis. Freudian dream-analysis, it might be argued, is impossible because we do not really know our dreams. We all too often notice after waking up that we have forgotten our dreams or that we can recall them only partly. What is more, there is no evidence that what we do remember is what we actually dreamt. Indeed, people who recall a dream and tell it to someone else frequently have the feeling that they are distorting the dream, that it was "somehow different." Does this not mean that the psychoanalytic interpretation of dreams is doomed from the outset?

Freud is aware of this objection, and he confronts it as follows. It is true, he says, that the psychoanalyst can work only with the dream as the dreamer remembers it and that, therefore, he will often work with distorted dreams. However, the distortions the psychoanalyst is faced with *are not random but follow the same pattern as the dream-work.* The forgetting and distorting that takes place after we have woken up is simply an additional process of censorship. (Freud does not provide a name for this process, but the phrase that suggests itself is *tertiary revision.*) In other words, the process that makes our dreams acceptable to our social conscience extends beyond our dreaming, continuing as it does to influence our ability to recall and recount what we dreamt. Hence, Freud concludes, the fact that the psychoanalyst has no direct access to the dreams he wishes to analyze is not a real problem. All it means is that he has to strip away an additional layer of the dreamer's self-deception.

The two objections discussed above both relate to the method of Freud's theory of dreams. But objections can also be raised with regard to its content, especially with regard to the central idea that dreams are disguised fulfillments of unconscious wishes. Is it really the case that all dreams are wish-fulfillments? Do people not dream frightening things too? Do they not have anxiety dreams, nightmares? Furthermore, how to explain dreams containing conscious wishes such as passing an exam or winning a football match? And what about blatantly sexual dreams, which, in the words of Ludwig Wittgenstein, are "common as rain"[9]?

In the case of anxiety dreams, the fear or discomfort is often on the manifest level only; the latent content still contains a wish-fulfillment. Additionally, such dreams may result from wish-fulfillments that went too far, or were about to go too far. The dreamer recoils from the extreme nature of his desires, and the dream turns scary. Finally, it is also possible that anxiety dreams are wish-fulfillments from start to finish. In this case, the wish that is being fulfilled is that of our social conscience wanting to punish us for our immoral deeds or desires.[10] Straightforward sexual dreams can be explained as the result of a failure on the part of the dream-work to do its job. The dream-work loses out against the overwhelming power of the drives and is no longer able to transform them into something decent.

Perhaps most difficult to explain are dreams that deal with the dreamer's everyday life, with his conscious wishes, his worries and fears, the things that happened to him on the day or days preceding the dream. How do these square with the idea that dreams are disguised fulfillments of unconscious wishes? Freud acknowledges that such dreams are frequent. But in his view our everyday wishes, worries, fears, and experiences merely provide a peg for the unconscious to hang its wishes on. Our everyday wishes and all the other things we experienced during the day may emerge again when we are dreaming, but the dream is not really about them. What the dream is about is our deepest and darkest desires; not the passing preoccupations of the day but the indestructible impulses of life itself.

In Freud's view the dream acts as a valve to the unconscious, reducing its pressure by providing it with a specific form of discharge. Like fantasies, art, and pornography, dreams are a compromise between acting out our drives and repressing them. Going out to kill and rape people is immoral and harmful to the victims; too much repression, too much pressure under the lid is unhealthy and harmful to ourselves. So we fantasize, we watch *Hamlet* or *Natural Born Killers*, we read *Playboy* — and we dream.

In other words, the dream helps us to cope with our innermost urges. In doing so, it sometimes weaves external stimuli such as the alarm clock going off or a car driving by into the dream story. But alarm clocks and cars are not the reason why we dream. In the same way, the dream sometimes integrates conscious wishes, worries, and other experiences from our waking lives. But these, too, are not the reason why we dream. They become part of the dream story either as a medium through which our drives can manifest themselves or because they are already bound up with our drives.

For example, there is no particular reason in itself why we should dream about a woman we saw on the bus or a difference of opinion we had with our boss. These are experiences we can deal with consciously; there is no need for a special mechanism like the dream to work them out of our system. It is only when our unconscious can attach itself to such experiences that they become relevant to the dream. Taking two clichéd examples, the woman on the bus may be woven into the dream story as a symbol for a cold and distant mother; the disagreement with our boss may act as a symbol for the relationship with our father. Alternatively, they may enter the dream because they themselves have a specific drive value for us; when we felt sexually attracted to the woman on the bus, for instance, or when she reminded us of someone whom we were close to in the past, or when the disagreement with our boss brought back unpleasant memories of a failed marriage.

Freud, then, is able to integrate even anxiety-dreams, straightforwardly sexual dreams, and dreams about our recent past and everyday preoccupations into his theory that every dream is the disguised fulfillment of an unconscious wish. Yet one may still wonder whether his theory is not too one-sided. Freud's basic assumption — that dreams provide us with a valve for relieving mental stress — is convincing enough. To follow on from this and assume that dreams also act as a valve to unconscious pressure seems convincing too. But to assume that dreams are *only* or *really* about unconscious pressure is considerably less convincing.

In fact, Freud himself feels somewhat uncomfortable about his general thesis and acknowledges that there are exceptions. To begin with, children's dreams often fulfill simple, straightforward wishes — going on holiday, eating strawberries, and the like — and do so virtually without distortion. They contain short and simple images that require no interpretation. Dreams stimulated by bodily needs such as hunger and thirst also satisfy conscious wishes in an undisguised manner. Thus we may dream of eating a lavish meal, or drinking water in great gulps. Then there are *Bequemlichkeitsträume,* dreams of convenience. They, too, are not about unconscious wishes and do not call for extensive analysis. Freud's account of this category is rather sketchy, but its defining characteristic seems to be the attempt to evoke a more comfortable life through the imaginary satisfaction of quasi-bodily needs and wishes. Examples include not wanting to get up and not having to get pregnant. Finally, in later years Freud came to believe that traumatic dreams — dreams that recall a severe mental shock — are not wish-fulfillments at all. For this category, though, he also ventured a possible counterargument. Such dreams might emanate from an unconscious desire to work through the trauma; that is, to come to terms with it by confronting it again and again.

Freud allows some exceptions to his dream theory, but he is at pains to minimize their importance. Indeed, in the concluding chapter of *Die Traumdeutung* he more or less ignores them. The inconsistency that results finds expression in such odd statements as: "we have constructed our theory of dreams on the assumption that the dream-wish which provides the motive power invariably originates from the unconscious — an assumption which, as I myself am ready to admit, cannot be proved to hold generally, though neither can it be rejected."[11]

The one-sidedness with which *Die Traumdeutung* focuses on the unconscious roots of the dream is at odds with the nature of psychoanalysis as a dynamic psychology.[12] According to Freud, the mind is an *interplay* of conscious and unconscious processes; and he rejects the charge of pansexualism — the accusation that psychoanalysis puts everything down to sex — by pointing out that it is not the inner sexual drives that determine our lives, but the conflicts (and their resolutions) between these drives and the demands of the outside world. Why then should dreams be more about our unconscious than about our conscious? And if there are dreams that are primarily manifestations of our unconscious drives, why can there not also be dreams which deal primarily with the outside world and our conscious attitude towards it? On the basis of Freud's general psychological theory, it would make more sense to view the dream as a mechanism that can deal both with our unconscious and our conscious, and to regard the extent to which it does the one or the other as a question which can only be answered with reference to individual dreams.

But what about Freud's argument that everyday experiences can be dealt with consciously and that, therefore, such experiences do not require special outlets such as those provided by dreams? To me, it seems that Freud is being overly rationalistic here. In theory, we may be able to handle our everyday experiences in a pragmatic and realistic manner; in practice, we almost invariably fail to do so. We worry about our exam results or our marriage, we are afraid of losing our jobs, we become angry when the man before us in the queue buys the last roll, we get all worked up when the central heating breaks down again; in short, we suffer from all sorts of conscious tension. Why then should the dream's therapeutic, pressure-reducing function be restricted to the unconscious? Why should the dream not provide an outlet for conscious tensions too?

Freud's view that the dream's real topics always come from the unconscious is problematic for another reason. It neglects both the frequency with which unconscious ideas become conscious and the gray area between conscious and unconscious mental processes. This neglect has its roots in Freud's general psychology. For although Freud acknowledges that what is unconscious can become conscious (it is, indeed, the main aim of psychoanalysis to achieve precisely this) and that what is conscious can become unconscious (namely, through repression), he tends to think of the relationship between consciousness and unconsciousness as something fairly stable. It seems to me, however, that in many cases what is conscious and what is unconscious alternate much more quickly than Freud assumes. Now Freud does not deny that such quick alternations are possible, but this possibility is not an integral part of his theory. The same holds true for the gray area between consciousness and unconsciousness. Freud does occasionally talk about drives within us whose existence we know of but refuse to acknowledge, but he does not integrate this semiconsciousness, or semi-unconsciousness, into his theory. If all this is true — if, in other words, the difference between consciousness and unconsciousness is much more relative than Freud's general theory would have it — then Freud's view that dreams are only or really about our unconscious has to be relativized as well.

Die Traumdeutung, then, is by no means an unproblematic book. But its value is not dependent on whether all dreams always fulfill unconscious wishes. What makes Freud's study of dreams important is the fact that it uncovers the influence of the unconscious on perfectly ordinary, everyday mental occurrences, experiences that are common to everyone. It provides a brilliant exemplification of the central psychoanalytic idea "that *what is suppressed continues to exist in normal people as well as ab-*

normal, and remains capable of mental functioning."[13] Far from merely introducing a new therapeutic technique, *Die Traumdeutung* helps us to gain a better understanding of *ourselves.*

The Interpretation of Freudian Slips I

Let us now turn to the second technique by which psychoanalysts try to gain access to the unconscious, the interpretation of Freudian slips. Freud himself, of course, does not use this term. He talks about *Fehlleistungen,* faulty actions or parapraxes (as the traditional English translation has it), actions that do not produce the desired result. Among the most common *Fehlleistungen* are slips of the pen and the tongue, the forgetting of names, words, and events, and the failure to carry out what one had planned to do. Freud's most extensive treatment of such slips and failures can be found in *Zur Psychopathologie des Alltagslebens* (The Psychopathology of Everyday Life, 1901), which despite its somewhat list-like appearance has become one of his most popular books.

The key idea behind Freud's concept of *Fehlleistungen* is that they are caused by the unconscious. They are not mere accidents, coincidences that cannot be explained, but the result of unconscious mental processes. We do not forget, overlook, and misspell by chance, but because our unconscious pressurizes us into doing so. This pressure can take many different forms and produce many different results. I wish to look at the most important ones. For the sake of clarity, I have divided them, perhaps somewhat artificially, into four categories.

The first category comprises those cases in which we forget something because unconsciously we do not wish to remember; that is, because the thing we are trying to remember has fallen victim to repression. Simple examples would be the inability to recollect the name of someone whom we have banished from our mind or the failure to retrieve traumatic experiences that we have suppressed. But this type of forgetting can also occur when the thing we are trying to remember is linked to or reminiscent of something we have repressed. One of the examples Freud mentions is that of an older widow, constantly trying to avoid memories of the days when she was younger, who is unable to recall the name of the psychiatrist Carl Gustav *Jung.* To take another example, Freud relates how he himself could at some point not come up with the name of the

Italian health resort Nervi, because as a psychiatrist he had quite enough to do with *Nerven* (nerves) anyway.

Into the second category fall those cases in which we forget something because unconsciously we wish to *avoid* an action we do not want to perform or to *make possible* an action we do want to perform. We forget about the train we have to catch because we do not really want to leave. We lose someone's telephone number because we do not feel like contacting him. We inadvertently leave our pen at a friend's flat because we want to see her again.[14] Now of course few cases are as simple to explain as these three. And as all of us constantly forget to do all sorts of things, we normally regard our omissions as mere accidents. However, such a view is too simple. This should be obvious from the fact that more often than not we benefit from these so-called chance events. As Freud points out, quoting his American translator A. A. Brill: "We are more apt to mislay letters containing bills than cheques."[15]

Often, the unconscious is only partially successful in getting its way. Instead of achieving the complete forgetting of a name, it only manages to distort it. Instead of making us think of sex, it only half succeeds in imposing itself upon us — so that suddenly we find ourselves saying "sex-backs" instead of "set-backs," or "masture" instead of "mature." These and similar slips constitute the third category of faulty actions. They represent a cross between our conscious thoughts and our unconscious wishes. Take the woman who says, "I am not domineering. My husband can do anything I want." Consciously, she does not want to dominate her husband; unconsciously, she does. The unconscious asserts its influence, triggering a slip of the tongue. The result is a statement midway between conscious thoughts (I do not dominate my husband) and unconscious wishes (my husband should do as I want). The same things happens when we remember, not the name we are trying to think of, but a substitute name. For instance, suppose Freud, instead of simply having forgotten the name of Nervi, had come up with something like Bervi. He would then have both remembered and not remembered; the substitute name would have been a trade-off between what he wanted to remember (Nervi) and what he wanted to forget (nerves). This is precisely the function of such compromise formations: to satisfy both our conscious and our unconscious.

Finally, the fourth category of faulty actions comprises those cases in which we fail to remember because the original memory of what happened has been replaced by another memory. Such replacements always take place in one direction only: important events are substituted by less important or even trivial ones. This happens when the original event is too traumatic, too painful, too embarrassing, or too "dirty" to be dealt with consciously. It then gets repressed and *covered*, as it were, by something more positive. Freud calls these substitute memories *Deckerinnerungen*, screen-memories.[16]

According to Freud, childhood memories in particular are prone to replacement. To take a somewhat extreme example, a woman who as a child was sexually abused by her father may remember, not this traumatic event, but how her father always wanted to hug her. The emotional aim of such substitutions is clear: to blanket a traumatic experience. What is less clear is why we should need replacement memories. Why do we not just repress traumatic experiences? Why cover them with something else? The reason seems to be that the power of some experiences is simply too strong; screen-memories then act as story frames which allow us to assimilate what we are not able to repress. In this sense, *Deckerinnerungen* resemble lightning conductors rather than screens or blankets.

There is an important difference between the fourth category of faulty actions and the other three. When we cannot come up with a name, lose someone's phone number, or make a slip of the tongue, then we know that something has gone awry. (Or when we do not notice the faulty action ourselves, someone usually points it out to us.) With screen-memories, we do *not* realize that something has gone wrong. In this sense, the fourth category is special. Still, the key characteristic of *Fehlleistungen* applies to all four categories: they are all bungled actions resulting, not from pure chance or conscious decisions, but from the pressure of the unconscious.

Because faulty actions result from the unconscious, they provide information about our deepest desires, our darkest obsessions, and our most strongly blocked-out memories. But this information cannot simply be read off. Like dreams, faulty actions require interpretation. Indeed, they often follow the same pattern as the dream-work. For example, substitute names are often linked to the real name in the same way that dream symbols are linked to dream-thoughts: by similarity (Bervi for

Nervi), pars pro toto (Brandt for Rembrandt), identity of function (Reagan for Kennedy), and so on. The interpretation of our slips is therefore as hazardous an enterprise as is the interpretation of our dreams. This does not invalidate *Fehlleistungen* as a way to gain access to the unconscious, but it does mean that a serious use of the concept cannot be as simple and straightforward as everyday psychologizing on the basis of "Freudian slips" may seem to suggest.

There is another problem we must look at. Perhaps even more than dreams, faulty actions raise the question as to what extent they actually emanate from *unconscious* wishes. The few examples given above already suggest that the exclusive link between faulty actions and unconscious wishes that Freud posits is unconvincing. Take the example of missing a train. The motive for this *may* be unconscious. But are there not also cases in which one misses a train while being conscious of the fact that one does not want to leave? I am not talking about cases in which one *deliberately* misses the train in order to be able to stay. I am talking about those cases in which one genuinely forgets (because one is engrossed in a conversation, for example) but, after the mistake has become apparent, immediately realizes that one does not really want to go. In such cases, the motive is not to be found in the unconscious, but in the preconscious.

As a matter of fact, many of the examples in *Zur Psychopathologie des Alltagslebens* are instances of faulty actions caused by pressure from the preconscious, rather than from the unconscious. The chairman who, on opening a particularly difficult meeting, declared it to be closed *knew* he dreaded the meeting and wished it to be over already; the man who suggested that a certain doctor should be insulted (instead of consulted) *knew* he respected the doctor's skills but disliked his manners; and so on. Freud seems to be so much in love with his examples that he does not realize that many of them do not support his key thesis. Indeed, *Zur Psychopathologie des Alltagslebens* even includes faulty actions that result from the clash between *conscious* thoughts, as in the following example that Freud borrowed from his Hungarian colleague Sándor Ferenczi.

> This reminds me of the *anecdeath* about . . ., I once wrote in my note-
> book. Of course I meant *anecdote;* the anecdote about a young gypsy
> who had been sentenced to death and who asked as a favour to be al-

lowed to choose the tree from which he was to be hanged. (In spite of a keen search, he failed to find any suitable tree.)[17]

Freud himself interprets Ferenczi's slip of the pen as resulting from impatience, surmising — quite reasonably — that when Ferenczi was about to write down the word "anecdote," he was already thinking of the gypsy who had been sentenced "to death." This, however, means that the slip resulted, not from an unconscious thought disturbing a conscious thought, but from one conscious thought disturbing another conscious thought.

Faulty actions, then, are caused not only by pressure from the unconscious, but also by pressure from the preconscious, and by clashes between different conscious thoughts; a fact, it should be added, that Freud eventually came to recognize himself.[18] But the situation is even more complicated than this. First, the distinctions among unconsciousness, preconsciousness, and consciousness are not absolute. As we observed in the previous section, what is conscious today may be unconscious tomorrow, and vice versa. Second — and this is something to which Freud himself alerts us — faulty actions can be overdetermined; that is, they can have more than one cause. Ferenczi's "anecdeath," for instance, may well have resulted from his thinking of the gypsy sentenced to death *and* from Ferenczi's harboring a death-wish against someone. When we put all this together, it becomes clear that the links between faulty actions and mental processes are both manifold and complex. Rather than simply expressing secret sexual wishes, as popular belief has it, "Freudian slips" reveal the fundamental diversity and ambiguity of the human mind.

The Interpretation of Freudian Slips II: Applications

Let us now have a closer look at some applications of the ideas examined above. To begin with, these ideas point to a way to gain access to a person's unconscious; they help the psychoanalyst to gather information of which the patient himself is not aware. This is the application which made us look at Freudian slips in the first place. As our discussion has shown, however, Freud's ideas can also be used to find out about a person's preconscious and conscious. The interpretation of faulty actions uncovers drives and desires on *all* mental levels — or, to avoid the misleading spatial metaphor, in all mental processes. What Freud says with regard to the influence of the unconscious can therefore with equal justice be applied to the influence of the preconscious and the conscious:

> He who has eyes to see and ears to hear becomes convinced that mortals can keep no secret. If their lips are silent, they gossip with their fingertips; betrayal forces its way through every pore.[19]

Faulty actions, then, point to hidden motives, to impulses, drives, and desires that we are not conscious of or that we do not want to acknowledge to ourselves or to others.[20] Some of these motives — say, not really wanting to leave — may be fairly innocent. Others, however, may not. Here, Freud's ideas acquire a critical edge. The attention to slips and instances of forgetting can help us to penetrate the innocuous surface of our actions and lay bare their other, darker dimensions. Do people work for charities because they wish to help other people, or are there also less altruistic reasons? Do people join the *Animal Liberation Front* because they want to put a stop to mink farming and similar activities, or do they have other motives too? Do people prevent a pedophile from living in their neighborhood because they are seeking to protect their children, or is there more to it? Of course, these questions are too complex to be dealt with on the basis of the concept of *Fehlleistungen* alone; their discussion requires a wider psychoanalytic framework. But faulty actions often provide important clues. Their interpretation is therefore a key element of psychoanalysis as a critical theory of society.

It is Freud himself who draws our attention to this wider use of psychoanalysis. One of the examples he mentions is eyewitness testimony. It is usually overlooked in court, he says, how often memories fall victim to unconsciously motivated forgetting. Society seems to think that swearing in a witness has some sort of purifying effect, but the influence of the unconscious cannot be removed by decree. Freud does not elaborate on this example but it is not hard to see its critical implications. After all, it is not only "normal" witnesses who may suffer from an inability to remember correctly, but also the police. An overzealous policeman may well forget about or overlook exonerating evidence, not because he wants to frame the accused (although this is known to happen as well) but because he is so focused on doing justice or making promotion that his unconscious tricks him into seeing only what incriminates the accused. The policeman then honestly believes he is doing a good job, for consciously he does not want to deceive. Unconsciously — that is, without being aware of it — he bends the law all the same.

We can take this example one step further. Freud's theory of faulty actions does not only alert us to the *possibility* of honest dishonesty; it also helps us to *identify* it. The interpretation of a slip of the tongue or the pen in a witness's statement allows us to look behind his intended meaning and seek out motives and inclinations of which he himself is not aware. Of course the theory can play a role in unmasking *conscious* deceit too. After all, faulty actions may also result from a clash between conscious processes. So when people say one thing (a lie) while they are simultaneously thinking of another (the truth), the tension between these mental contents may well produce revealing slips.[21]

Another example of a wider use of psychoanalysis that Freud mentions is concerned with historiography, the way a people remembers and describes its past. National memories, Freud says, often follow the same pattern as the memories of individuals. Both are subject to various forms of unintentional but "useful" forgetting, and in both cases painful events are often blanketed by less painful ones. National myths and legends, all too often even official histories, leave out, overemphasize, paper over, and play down. To illustrate Freud's view with a modern example, Britain remembers its heroic stance in the Second World War but tends to forget its senseless bombardment of Dresden. Similarly, Dutch national memory still sees the war crimes committed by the Dutch army in Indonesia (in the late 1940s, when Indonesia was still a Dutch colony) in terms of necessary police actions tainted only by the occasional transgressions of a few individuals. As with the faulty actions of an individual, all this is not due to a deliberate strategy; it happens without a people being aware of it. And as with individuals, nations may give themselves away by slips — strange inconsistencies, revealing gaps, and involuntary admissions — in what they remember; that is, in their national histories, literary canons, and the like.

The final application I wish to look at takes us to the field of literature. The psychoanalytic view of faulty actions, Freud says, is not completely original. In affairs of love, people have always felt that forgetting is more than simply "forgetting." A man who forgets a date with his girlfriend will usually apologize in vain. "She will not fail to reply: 'A year ago you wouldn't have forgotten. You evidently don't care for me any longer.' Even if he should . . . try to excuse his forgetfulness by pleading pressure of business, the only outcome would be that the lady . . . would reply: 'How curious that business distractions like these never turned up in the past!'"[22] Some scholars too, says Freud, have suspected that there is more to forgetfulness than meets the eye. By way of example, he quotes the philosopher Friedrich Nietzsche: "*I did this,* says my Memory. *I cannot have done this,* says my Pride and remains inexorable. In the end — Memory yields."[23]

It is creative writers, however, who according to Freud have shown the deepest intuitive insights into unconscious motivation. That is why the theory of faulty actions is relevant to the study of literature. It can reveal aspects of a literary character that psychologically less sensitive interpretations tend to miss out on. Let us take a look at two examples from *Zur Psychopathologie des Alltagslebens.*

The first is one that Freud borrowed from his colleague Otto Rank. In Shakespeare's *The Merchant of Venice,* Portia is forced by her father to marry the man who chooses correctly among three different caskets. After several wrong choices made by men she does not like, it is now Bassanio's turn, the man she loves. As the election of her husband is dependent on his picking the right casket, she cannot confess her love to Bassanio before he has made the right choice. Yet this is precisely what she would like to do. At first, she manages to stay within the bounds of what is expected of her by just telling Bassanio that she likes him and wants him to stay a little longer.

> I pray you tarry, pause a day or two
> Before you hazard, for in choosing wrong
> I lose your company; therefore forbear a while, —
> There's something tells me (but it is not love)
> I would not lose you. . . .[24]   (3.2.1–5)

But her suppressed desire to tell Bassanio the truth — that she does love him and wants to marry him — exerts its influence and within seconds produces a slip of the tongue revealing her true feelings:

> They [i.e., your eyes] have o'erlook'd me and divided me,
> One half of me is yours, the other half yours, —
> Mine own I would say. . . . (3.2.15–17)

Portia tries to comply with her father's wishes, and to this end misrepresents her feelings; "it is not love," she says. But her own wishes will not be denied completely. The result is a slip through which it becomes apparent what she really feels for Bassanio: that, as far as she is concerned, she is his already.

The second example, which Freud also borrowed from a colleague, concerns *The Island Pharisees,* a novel by John Galsworthy, winner of the 1932 Nobel Prize for Literature. The example runs as follows.

> A very instructive and transparent example of the sureness with which imaginative writers know how to employ the mechanism of parapraxes . . . in the psychoanalytic sense is contained in John Galsworthy's novel *The Island Pharisees.* The story centres round the vacillations of a young man of the well-to-do middle-class between his strong social sympathy and the conventional attitudes of his class. Chapter XXVI portrays the ways in which he reacts to a letter from a young ne'er-do-well, to whom — prompted by his original attitude to life — he had supplied help on two or three occasions. The letter contains no direct request for money, but paints a picture of great distress which can have no other meaning. Its recipient at first rejects the idea of throwing the money away on a hopeless case instead of using it to support charitable causes. "To give a helping hand, a bit of himself, a nod of fellowship to any fellow-being irrespective of a claim, merely because he happened to be down, was sentimental nonsense! The line must be drawn! But in the muttering of this conclusion he experienced a twinge of honesty. 'Humbug! You don't want to part with your money, that's all!'"
>
> Thereupon he wrote a friendly letter, ending with the words: "I enclose a cheque. Yours sincerely, Richard Shelton."
>
> "Before he had written out the cheque, a moth fluttering round the candle distracted his attention, and by the time he had caught and put it out he had forgotten that the cheque was not enclosed." The letter was posted in fact just as it was.
>
> There is however an even subtler motivation for the lapse of memory than the break-through of the selfish purpose, which had apparently been surmounted, of avoiding giving away the money.

At the country seat of his future parents-in-law, surrounded by his fiancée, her family and their guests, Shelton felt isolated; his parapraxis indicates that he longed for his protégé who, as a result of his past and his view of life, forms a complete contrast to the irreproachable company, uniformly moulded by one and the same set of conventions, that surround him. And in fact this person, who can no longer keep his place without being supported, does in fact arrive some days later to get an explanation of why the promised cheque was not there.[25]

At first sight, this psychoanalytic interpretation may seem far-fetched. Indeed, when the young vagabond (his name is Ferrand) finally arrives, the novel states that Shelton "cursed the young man's coming."[26] But the interpretation ties in with other observations. Shelton's releasing the moth, for example, points to an unconscious desire to escape his conventional surroundings; similar motives occur throughout the novel. His deliberations, too, hint at unconscious thoughts. The phrase "to help someone, because he happened to be down," written in free indirect speech, is ambiguous; the "he" can refer both to Ferrand and to Shelton himself. These examples make it clear that the novel aims to bring out — obliquely — the fact that Shelton is unaware of the complexity of his motivations.[27] It is this compatibility with other features of the text that makes the psychoanalytic interpretation of Shelton's forgetfulness plausible.

Freud's explanation of faulty actions is only one of his many ideas that are relevant to the study of literature. The concepts of repression and projection, for instance, can be applied in similar ways. But there is more. Psychoanalysis not only provides a conceptual framework that helps us to discover and interpret things in literary texts that the writer has deliberately put there; its concepts do not only enable us to talk about texts as embodiments of a great writer's psychological insights. Psychoanalysis *also* provides a conceptual framework that helps us to discover and interpret things in literary texts that the writer himself *does not know are in there;* that is, it enables us to talk about literary texts as embodiments of a writer's *unconscious motivations.* A writer's mind, like any other human being's, is made up of conscious, preconscious, and unconscious mental processes, and what he does, says, or writes results from the interplay between these processes.

Thus, the relevance of psychoanalysis to the study of literature stretches far beyond the analysis of the feelings and actions of *literary characters*. Freud's ideas also enable us to analyze the *writer's* mental processes. Moreover, as every literary text is the result of the interplay of its author's conscious, preconscious, and unconscious mental processes, psychoanalysis can tell us something about the *literary text* itself, about its structure and meaning. All this will be discussed in detail in part 2.

The Interpretation of Free Associations

The third technique psychoanalysts use to gain access to the unconscious is the interpretation of free associations. What are free associations, and how are they linked to the unconscious? As we have seen, when asking patients about their symptoms Freud would invariably encounter a particular difficulty. The closer he got to the core of the patients' repressions, the stronger their (unconscious) resistance became. And the more Freud insisted, the less productive the sessions became. His patients would unwittingly begin to give indefinite answers, equivocate, or go off on a tangent. So Freud decided to reverse the approach. Instead of seeking to direct his patients' thoughts, he allowed, indeed encouraged, the patients to let their thoughts wander off. He simply asked them to focus on a particular symptom and to tell him everything and anything that came into their heads. He stressed that they should really tell him *all* they happened to think of, even the things that seemed trivial or meaningless, and that they should not try to remain focused on the symptom, or to be consistent, but that they should let their thoughts run freely. In this way, one thought would trigger another, which would trigger yet another thought, and so on. Freud called these spontaneously produced and interconnected thoughts *free associations*.

The idea behind this new approach was this. Freud had come to realize that the more his patients were able to relax and let go, the weaker was their resistance.[28] And the weaker their resistance was, the more easily the content of their unconscious could manifest itself. So everything his patients said in this relaxed and unfocused way had to be closely linked to their unconscious. The meanderings of their free associations were thus not random and meaningless but, on the contrary, directed by their unconscious. If interpreted correctly, these free associations could therefore lead the psychoanalyst to the unconscious origins of his patients' problems.

Against this backdrop, it becomes apparent that the phrase *free associations* is misleading. It is not the case that the patients consciously and intentionally link up specific ideas. They do not associate in the same way that they calculate sums or do crosswords. Rather, their associating is something over which they have no control, something which happens to them. Therefore, Freud's own phrase — *freie Einfälle* — is much better than the English translation, highlighting as it does the passive nature of the process. (*Etwas fällt mir ein* means "something occurs to me.") But even the German phrase is misleading. For the so-called *freie Einfälle* are anything but free; they are, after all, determined by the unconscious.

Free associations do not bring up the unconscious material itself but merely provide hints at it. That is why interpretation is necessary. Let me illustrate this difficult but important point. Suppose a man is being unfaithful to his wife. In order to hide this from her he will seek to evade potentially embarrassing questions, avoid "dangerous" topics of conversation, and do everything to convince his wife that he still loves her. He will, for instance, say that he is busy with an important project and needs to work overtime; he will try to steer the conversation away from adultery and related topics; he will stress as if in passing that he is not "into" redheads (his girlfriend has red hair); he will tell his wife more often than before how much he loves her; and so on. At a superficial glance, the things he says seem unconnected. Yet they all have their origin in his attempt to allay his wife's suspicion. They are all ways to get away from the issue of his adultery.

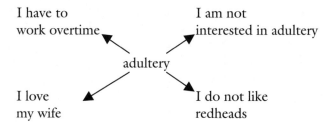

However, precisely because the things he says are directed by what he is trying to hide, they all point to one and the same thing. Although not themselves expressions of his adultery, they hint at it. If his wife links them up and interprets them correctly, she will have little difficulty in discovering what lies behind them.

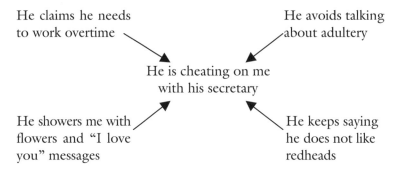

The interpretation of free associations works in the same way. Of course, unlike the protestations of the man in our example, free associations are not determined by the patient's conscious mental processes but by his unconscious mental processes. But like the adulterer's protestations, they are determined by a hidden agency and are therefore centered around a hidden core. Like the adulterer's protestations, they seem unconnected and yet hint at a specific mental attitude of the person who produces them. And like the adulterer's protestations they put the critical listener on the track of what lies behind them.

Obviously, the interpretation of free associations is no easy matter. Psychoanalysts therefore combine it with other techniques such as the interpretation of a patient's dreams and faulty actions. This we have looked at already: using more than one technique allows the psychoanalyst to carry out an internal consistency check on his interpretations, and to modify or correct them accordingly. However, the interpretation of free associations is not only useful as an *addition* to the interpretation of dreams and the interpretation of faulty actions; it can also be used as *part* of these other techniques. If, say, the psychoanalyst is unable to interpret a particular dream element, he can ask the patient to associate on it. Starting off from this dream element, the patient's *Einfälle* (the things that occur to him, that well up from his mind) will then, if interpreted correctly, assume a pattern that leads the psychoanalyst to the unconscious thoughts behind it.

Associating, then, plays an important role in the psychoanalyst's attempt to circumvent his patients' resistance and gain access to their unconscious. This does not imply that free association is simply the opposite of resistance. When people associate, the process of repression is weaker than usual, but it is not inactive. If it were, the unconscious contents themselves, not just hints at them, would emerge. Even in dreams (that is, at a time when people are even more relaxed than when they are associating) processes of repression, of pushing back and censoring, are operative. In their own way, free associations — the seemingly random route they take, their apparent unconnectedness, their frequently trivial or meaningless appearance — are expressions of resistance too. Neither does the importance of free association imply that resistance is nothing but an obstacle to the psychoanalyst. On the contrary, the process of resistance may contain important indications as to what mental contents are being held back. The psychoanalyst will therefore try to interpret both his patients' free associations *and* their more direct attempts at resistance.

The Interpretation of Resistance and Transference

Indefinite answers, equivocations, denials, the avoidance of topics, vagueness — these are all means by which people resist the psychoanalyst's attempts to penetrate their unconscious. To be sure, people are not aware that this is what they are doing; they think they are being as honest and helpful as they possibly can. It is their unconscious which tricks them into being evasive, makes them consider a particular topic irrelevant, and leads them to believe that the psychoanalyst is talking nonsense. In this sense, it is the unconscious itself that puts up a resistance against the psychoanalyst. But precisely because this is so, resistance not only impedes psychoanalytic understanding but also facilitates it. Because resistance is produced by the unconscious, it can lead the psychoanalyst to the unconscious. That is why the interpretation of resistance, after the interpretation of dreams, faulty actions, and free associations, is the fourth major means by which psychoanalysts try to gain access to the unconscious.

In order to interpret his patients' resistance, the psychoanalyst will ask such questions as: what are the topics they are trying to avoid; which ideas do they deny with conspicuous vehemence; why are they suddenly talking in generalities? There is, however, one form of resistance that requires different questions, because it is linked less to the *issues* the psychoanalyst and the patient talk about than to the *relationship* between psychoanalyst and patient. This form of resistance is known as *Übertragung*, transference.

By *transference* Freud means any form of displacement carried out by the patient and directed at the psychoanalyst. Displacement, we noted in the section on dreams, is the unconscious transfer of an idea concerning one person onto another. Transference can therefore be defined, in the words of the psychoanalyst and Freud biographer Peter Gay, as "the patient's way, sometimes subtle and often blatant, of [unconsciously] endowing the analyst with [real or imagined] qualities that properly belong to beloved (or hated) persons, past and present, in the 'real' world."[29]

As with displacement, transference may involve the transfer of both positive and negative ideas. In the first case, it leads to an overvaluation of the psychoanalyst's qualities, to an affectionate devotion towards him combined with jealousy of people close to him, or even to (platonic or sexual) love. In the second case, it leads to contempt for the psychoanalyst and to aggression and hatred towards him. Why should transference take place? What lies behind it? The answer can be found in the concept of resistance. All people are continually subject to two unconscious processes: pressure from the unconscious trying to manifest itself on the one hand, repression pushing back the contents of the unconscious on the other. If a psychoanalyst attempts to gain entrance to their unconscious, the repressive process will become stronger and they will start putting up resistance. One of the forms this resistance can take is transference: instead of bringing his unconscious emotional life into consciousness, the patient re-experiences it in his relation to the psychoanalyst. That is why the psychoanalyst is suddenly a powerful and learned man (as the patient's father was or as the patient wished him to be), or a good friend (as the patient's brother was or as the patient thought he was), or an uncaring tyrant (as the patient's boss is either in reality or in the eyes of the patient). The patient has projected qualities of persons from his emotional life onto the psychoanalyst.

Thus, patients will begin to look upon and behave towards the psychoanalyst as if he were their father, brother, boss, and so on. Such transferences and transference-induced actions may be triggered by particular questions or issues that arise during a session, but they can also emerge quite independently. For example, if the patient is a young vulnerable woman and the psychoanalyst a fatherly man, there is a fair chance that she will want to be treated as a beloved daughter, irrespective of the things the two of them happen to be talking about. Moreover, relationships based on transference (like other relationships) usually develop their own internal dynamics. Paying attention to the questions or issues under discussion will therefore not, or only to a limited degree, help the psychoanalyst to turn this particular form of resistance to his advantage. How, then, is he to make analytic capital out of the phenomenon of transference?

Transference may be exploited in three different ways. First, it usually begins as positive (affectionate) transference and as such facilitates the analytic process. The patient will want to please the psychoanalyst, to help him as best as he can, to show himself worthy of him, and so on. By shrewdly playing to this state of mind the psychoanalyst can achieve things that otherwise would have been beyond his reach. Second, the power that the psychoanalyst now holds enables him to re-educate the patient to a certain degree. For example, if the psychoanalyst is looked upon as a father, he can try to undo the educational mistakes made by the patient's real father. This procedure is not, admittedly, without its risks. His power may tempt the psychoanalyst into re-creating the patient in his own image, thus unwittingly undermining the patient's individuality. Re-education can only be successful if the psychoanalyst manages the paradoxical task of influencing the patient in such a way that the patient achieves greater independence. The third way in which transference may be exploited is the most important one. *Transference can be interpreted as an expression of the patient's unconscious emotional life and thus lead the psychoanalyst to the unconscious roots of his patient's problems.* Instead of remembering, the patient acts out parts of what he has repressed and in doing so provides important clues to what occupies his unconscious mind.

Using the phenomenon of transference to good effect is not easy. Like the interpretation of dreams, faulty actions, and free associations, the interpretation of transference is a highly complex and uncertain enterprise. There are other difficulties too. We said that transference usually begins as positive (affectionate) transference, but it *may* also begin as negative (hostile) transference. Moreover, at some point positive transference almost inevitably changes over into transference of the negative variety. In fact, transference is always ambivalent. Positive transference always also comprises negative elements; negative transference always also comprises positive elements. In this respect, relationships based on transference are like any other relationship. There is no admiration without repressed envy, no devotion without repressed aggression, no love without repressed hatred. When the patient's exaggerated expectations are frustrated (which is bound to happen, since the psychoanalyst is not all-powerful, cannot have an exclusive relationship with a particular patient, cannot grant his patient's sexual wishes, and so on), his repressed hostility will come to the surface. In other words, sooner or later the psychoanalyst will be faced with a patient who hates him, who becomes aggressive towards him, who thinks he is a quack. This is a serious difficulty for both of them. It makes things difficult for the psychoanalyst because the patient is no longer cooperative and trusting; it makes things difficult for the patient because he does not view the situation as a reflection of his past but as a new problem in the present. Only when the psychoanalyst manages to convince the patient that what is happening is not the emergence of genuine feelings within the analytic situation, but a surfacing of repressed emotional elements from outside the analytic situation, can this obstacle be removed.

There is yet another difficulty the psychoanalyst has to overcome if he is to turn the phenomenon of transference to his advantage. It is not only patients but also the psychoanalyst himself who may fall victim to transference. Confronted with his patients' admiration, affection, or love (or, alternatively, their contempt, aggression, or hatred), he may start to project positive or negative ideas onto *them*. This type of transference — transference carried out by the psychoanalyst and directed at the patient — is called *Gegenübertragung,* counter-transference. So the psychoanalyst needs to convince himself, too, that the patient is not really an admiring pupil, not really the son or daughter he always wanted, not really someone who is in love with him. Even more than the interpretation of dreams, faulty actions and free associations, the interpretation of transference requires that the psychoanalyst should preserve his objectivity and not lose himself in the vortex of the emotions generated by the analysis. Of all four techniques to gain access to the unconscious, the interpretation of transference therefore provides perhaps the greatest challenge to the practicing psychoanalyst.

Notes

[1] After having been obliged to dismiss his servant Lampe, who had served him for many years, the philosopher Immanuel Kant put a note on his desk saying "Lampe must be forgotten!" The result was predictable.

[2] Sigmund Freud, *The Interpretation of Dreams,* trans. James Strachey, ed. Angela Richards, vol. 4 of *The Penguin Freud Library,* ed. Angela Richards and Albert Dickson (Harmondsworth: Penguin, 1991), 244.

[3] Freud explains this type of symbolism, which according to him can also be found in mythology and folklore, as part of mankind's psychocultural heritage. However, regardless of whether such universal symbolism exists or not, the fact remains that it is reductive to assume that any symbol can have only one, predetermined meaning.

[4] Freud, *Interpretation of Dreams,* 531.

[5] Freud, *Interpretation of Dreams,* 531–32.

[6] Freud, *Interpretation of Dreams,* 630; the allusion is to the poem "Zu fragmentarisch ist Welt und Leben!" in Heinrich Heine's *Die Heimkehr* (Homecoming, 1826).

[7] Freud, *Interpretation of Dreams,* 769.

[8] Sigmund Freud, *Five Lectures on Psychoanalysis,* in *Two Short Accounts of Psycho-Analysis,* trans. and ed. James Strachey (Harmondsworth: Penguin, 1977), 60.

[9] Ludwig Wittgenstein, *Lectures & Conversations on Aesthetics, Psychology and Religion,* ed. Cyril Barrett (Oxford: Blackwell, 1966), 47.

[10] This is perhaps easier to understand against the backdrop of Freud's tripartite model of the mind (ego/superego/id). A detailed treatment of this model is offered in chapter 3.

[11] Freud, *Interpretation of Dreams,* 757; translation modified. The Penguin translation endeavors to minimize the confusion by rendering *zurückweisen* (reject) as *disprove.*

[12] From a historical perspective, the focus is of course understandable enough: Freud sought to provide a counterweight to the many neurologists and psychiatrists who neglected the role of the unconscious.

[13] Freud, *Interpretation of Dreams,* 768; translation modified.

[14] Here, Freud quotes his British colleague Ernest Jones, who remarks half-jokingly that one "can almost measure the success with which a physician is practising therapy" by "the size of the collection of umbrellas, handkerchiefs, purses, and so on that he could make in a month" (*The Psychopathology of Everyday Life,* trans. Alan Tyson, ed. Angela Richards, vol. 5 of *The Penguin Freud Library,* ed. Angela Richards and Albert Dickson [Harmondsworth: Penguin, 1991], 273).

[15] Freud, *Psychopathology,* 211.

[16] It should be added that, according to Freud, *Deckerinnerungen* do not only cover events that actually took place; sometimes it is wishes or fantasies that are replaced.

[17] Freud, *Psychopathology,* 174; translation modified.

[18] An extensive discussion of faulty actions that reflects this more differentiated view can be found in Freud's *Vorlesungen zur Einführung in die Psychoanalyse* (Introductory Lectures on Psychoanalysis, 1917), trans. James Strachey, ed. James Strachey and Angela Richards, vol. 1 of *The Penguin Freud Library,* ed. Angela Richards and Albert Dickson (Harmondsworth: Penguin, 1991), 50–108. As in the case of *Die Traumdeutung,* Freud's original one-sided focus on the unconscious can be explained from his desire to oppose the prevailing scientific tendency to reduce mental phenomena to conscious or biological processes.

[19] Sigmund Freud, *Case Histories I,* trans. Alix and James Strachey, ed. Angela Richards, vol. 8 of *The Penguin Freud Library,* ed. Angela Richards and Albert Dickson (Harmondsworth: Penguin, 1990), 114, as translated in Peter Gay, *Freud: A Life for Our Time* (New York/London: W. W. Norton, 1988), xix.

[20] I leave aside the straightforward case in which we are both aware of the root of our slip and willing to tell other people about it.

[21] Obviously, this method should not be applied uncritically. Faulty actions do not necessarily reveal what a person really did. They point to mental preoccupations, and these may include worries and fantasies.

[22] Freud, *Psychopathology,* 205.

[23] Freud, *Psychopathology,* 198; the quotation is from *Jenseits von Gut und Böse* (Beyond Good and Evil, 1886), 4:68.

[24] William Shakespeare, *The Merchant of Venice,* ed. John Russell Brown, The Arden Shakespeare (London: Methuen, 1961).

[25] Freud, *Psychopathology,* 182–83.

[26] John Galsworthy, *The Island Pharisees* (1904; London: Heinemann, 1927), 230.

[27] When after some time Ferrand decides to leave, Shelton's reaction is described as "a curious mingling of relief, regret, goodwill" (Galsworthy, *The Island Pharisees,* 248).

[28] Here we may recall what was observed with regard to dreams. When people are less worried about the outside world, their need to push back the contents of the unconscious is less strong; hence their resistance is weaker.

[29] Gay, *Freud: A Life for Our Time,* 253.

3: The Unconscious and Society

THE PRECEDING CHAPTERS HAVE uncovered something I have not yet been able to explain, the contradictory nature of the unconscious. For example, we observed that dreams can satisfy *both* unconscious sensual wishes *and* the unconscious desire of our social conscience to punish us for deeds and desires it considers immoral. More importantly, on several occasions we made the observation that people are simultaneously subject to unconscious pressure from sensual wishes striving for satisfaction and to unconscious counter-pressure in the form of a repression process pushing these wishes back. These observations show that the unconscious is not unified, but split; that it consists of different types of wishes, of drives pushing in different directions, of different *conative trends*. (The Latin verb *conari* means "strive for.")

How are these different conative trends to be accounted for? Where do they come from? Freud's original, dualistic, model of the mind left this open, distinguishing merely between unconsciousness and consciousness (and preconsciousness). It was only later, in the 1920s, that Freud managed to fill the gap with a more subtle theory, the tripartite model of the mind.[1]

Id, Ego, and Superego I

As the term indicates, the tripartite model of the mind posits *three* different mental agencies: the id (*das Es*),[2] the ego (*das Ich*), and the superego (*das Über-Ich*).

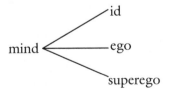

The id constitutes the lustful, aggressive (in Freud's terminology, sexual) part of our personality. It comprises both the pleasure-seeking urges with which we are born and the wishes, obsessions, and other affects derived from or associated with them. It is not a region of the mind, but a process made up of drives which are always operative, constantly pushing for satisfaction and constantly being pushed back (repression), diverted into cultural activities (sublimation), acted out (temporary satisfaction), or discharged in other ways (dreams, faulty actions). The id does not argue or deliberate, possesses no values or rules, and respects neither common sense nor logic. It is pure craving. As our id-drives usually remain repressed, finding expression only in short-lived and apparently unconnected actions, the true nature of this part of our personality remains in the dark. Freud therefore describes the id as being *unconscious.*

The superego comprises the norms, values, and ideals that upbringing and education have instilled in us. It is not equivalent to our conscience, however, as it does not simply coincide with our conscious and preconscious ethics. Having its origins in childhood, it contains many elements that we are no longer aware of and that are not relevant or appropriate to our current lives. These unconscious injunctions may well be in conflict with our current ethics but on an unconscious level continue to influence us all the same. This is apparent from the guilt we can feel about actions which we rationally do not consider to have been wrong. That is why Freud says "that the normal man is not only far more immoral than he believes but also far more moral than he knows."[3] Finally, although the superego is a more socially oriented agency than the id, it is not more benevolent, rational, or considerate. In its own way, it is just as selfish, pushing for ethical perfection in the same uncompromising manner that the id pushes for erotic pleasure.

Whereas the id and the superego strive for immediate satisfaction without regard for the well-being of the person as a whole, the ego seeks to achieve compromises. The id represents an unconscious pressure on us to live in complete accordance with our own innermost wishes; the superego represents an unconscious pressure on us to live in complete accordance with the wishes that other people (first and foremost our parents and teachers) have instilled in us; and the ego tries to find a healthy *balance* between our own wishes and those of others. Additionally, the ego is engaged in the interaction with the outside world. It needs to manage a host of social relations involving different people, different types of dependence, and varying degrees of emotional involvement. In brief, the ego faces a threefold challenge: "from the external world, from the libido of the id, and from the severity of the superego."[4]

The ego is more than the conscious and preconscious personality. It not only thinks, feels, worries, knows, learns, remembers, and fantasizes; it also *represses, resists, projects,* and so on. These operations are unconscious: we are not aware of the fact that we are performing them, and we have no control over them. The ego's unconscious defense mechanisms are therefore just as blind and irrational as the drives of the id and superego.

The ego, then, has at its disposal both "realistic problem-solving methods," and "methods that deny, falsify, or distort reality," as Calvin Hall puts it.[5] This does not mean that the former are always preferable to the latter. If we did not repress some very real and dangerous urges, we would turn into perverts. If our unconscious defense system did not on occasion embellish the truth a little, we would become completely overwhelmed by feelings of guilt and frustration about the many mistakes and weaknesses that are the inevitable result of man's imperfection. Being neither supermen nor robots, we need our unconscious defense mechanisms just as much as we need our conscious fantasies. On the other hand, placing too much reliance on unconscious coping strategies is an impediment to personal growth. This, unfortunately, is the rule rather than the exception. People have a tendency to take the easy way out, and to resist any attempt to confront them with the nasty facts they have repressed. This is harmful not just to them but all too often to others as well. And as long as reality is not acknowledged, nothing will change. That is why psychoanalysis seeks to bring into consciousness as many counterproductive ego, id, and superego processes as is realistically possible. Its main aim is what Freud calls *"education to reality."*[6]

Two further remarks are in order. For one thing, the internal pressure created by unconscious drives and the external pressure emanating from the outside world are always interrelated. Both the id and the superego seek to influence not just our mental state but the way we deal with the world around us; and our attempts to adapt to or gain mastery over the environment affect our drives (abstinence leads to sexual frustration, crimes provoke the superego, and so on). For another, it is not the case that the id always pulls us in just one direction, and the superego always in one other direction. Rather, the id may pull in different directions at the same time. This happens for example when a person harbors both unconscious feelings of love and unconscious feelings of hatred towards someone. The superego, too, can influence us in different directions at the same time. If an unemployed single mother swindles the insurance company in order to pay for her children's education, her superego may make her feel both good (because she is helping her children) and bad (because she is committing a crime).

Before moving on, we must briefly look at a problem raised by this new theory of the mind. In the dualistic model, the conscious and the unconscious were seen as mental agencies. In the tripartite model, by contrast, they are viewed as qualities of mental agencies: the conscious part of the ego, the unconscious processes of the id, and so forth. They are transformed from nouns into adjectives, so to speak. But although this makes the relationship between consciousness and unconsciousness more sophisticated, it does not completely remove the dualism of the older model. The new theory, too, distinguishes strictly between conscious and unconscious mental states and treats their relationship as being more or less stable. This is most clearly to be seen from Freud's definition of the id as an unconscious process. The tripartite model of the mind, then, is vulnerable to the same twofold charge as its predecessor: it ignores that what is conscious and what is unconscious may alternate relatively quickly, and that there are varying degrees of consciousness and unconsciousness.

Id, Ego, and Superego II: Three Examples

Freud's tripartite model of the mind is a sophisticated instrument that provides genuine insight into the complexity of mental processes. As this analytic potential may not be immediately apparent, I wish to illustrate it with three examples.

To begin with, the model does not consider the "dark" drives of the id as what is bad in us, nor the social norms, values, and ideals we have internalized — the superego — as what is good in us. The id motivates us to seek sensual pleasure; the superego motivates us to behave socially.

Both are conducive to our mental and physical health. Sensual pleasure is agreeable in itself, and social obedience contributes to our living together in an agreeable way. In this sense, our superego is not better than our id, nor our id better than our superego. Problems only arise when there is an imbalance between the two; that is, when one suppresses the other. This ethical impartiality of Freud's model makes it possible to bring out the complexity of the relationship between psychology and morality, in particular the potential psychological badness of moral goodness, and the potential psychological goodness of moral badness. How is this to be understood?

Both the id and the superego, I said above, strive for immediate satisfaction without regard for the well-being of the person as a whole. In the case of the superego this means that we are impelled to live *in total obedience* to the social rules we have internalized. The superego is an absolutist. It accepts no transgression, however small, no slip-up, however accidental, no exception, however temporary, no compromise, however well-intentioned. Moreover, to the superego *thinking* of crossing the line is just as bad as actually *doing* it. To put it in biblical terms, the superego rules according to the maxim expressed by Jesus in the Sermon on the Mount: "Ye have heard that it was said by them of old time, Thou shalt not commit adultery: But I say unto you, That whosoever looketh on a woman to lust after her hath committed adultery with her already in his heart." And if we do sin (to retain the biblical vocabulary), the superego is quick to punish us by making us feel bad, guilty, weak, or inadequate.

This explains what the psychological badness of moral goodness consists in: if we try to be *too* good, we shall be punished by our superego and become unhappy. For none of us is perfect; we are all "sinners." Only saints can live like saints (and usually they do not manage either). From a psychoanalytic perspective, therefore, moral goodness is good only up to a point; the demands of the superego always need to be counterbalanced by those of the id and relativized by the ego's acceptance of man's imperfection.

People driven predominantly by their superego are faced with three problems. Their superego always demands more than they can deliver; it forces them to evaluate the result of their actions in too critical a way; and it produces a strong sense of guilt every time they do not live up to its inflated demands. Such people constantly suffer from the feeling that they are bad. They become disgusted with themselves and often fall into a depression. As Freud puts it:

> Experience teaches us that for most people there is a limit beyond which their constitution cannot comply with the demands of civilization. All who wish to be more noble-minded than their constitution allows fall victims to neurosis; they would have been more healthy if it could have been possible for them to be less good.[7]

There is another possible reaction to an overly strong superego: not depression (and perhaps suicide), but ruthless activism (and perhaps murder). Because of its absolutist nature, the superego is never satisfied; everything and anything that it does not consider perfect is considered bad. The superego's world-view is rigidly dualistic: something is either good or bad, with nothing in between. Since in reality things are always a mixture of good and bad, or good from one perspective and bad from another, people driven predominantly by their superego cannot but believe the whole world, and not just their own thoughts and deeds, to be entirely bad. The outcome is either a depression ("there is no future," "everything is going down the drain") *or a radical desire to do away with things as they are and wipe the slate clean.* The absolute goodness that the superego demands but which is nowhere to be found in reality is then not seen as unattainable but gets transposed onto the future. It becomes a goal one needs to work towards. For anyone with such a mindset, moreover, an acceptance of the world's rules and conventions would entail complicity in its badness. Any means to achieve the utopian end of total goodness is therefore considered justified. This is the psychological stuff that many terrorists and revolutionaries are made of.

Against this backdrop it becomes clear, not only why moral goodness can be psychologically bad (and can result in morally bad behavior such as terrorism), but also why moral badness can be psychologically good. A little bit of evil may restore the balance between id and superego and thus reduce a tension that otherwise might lead to a much stronger explosion of id-forces. For example, relationships in which both partners manage to behave selfishly from time to time are usually happier than relationships in which the partners are always trying to be nice to each other. People who swallow everything down are generating so much internal pressure that they either become unhappy or ultimately "blow a fuse." In this sense, living is like being on a diet. Occasional small sins may help to prevent the big attack of gluttony that so often ruins the whole diet. Socially, the least harmful way to satisfy our id-drives is obviously by various types of fantasies: dreams and daydreams, literature, film, and so on. That is why, from a psychoanalytic point of view, the banning of pornography is not necessarily cultural progress. For it is to be feared that the fewer vicarious methods of satisfaction the id has, the more easily it will turn to real ones.

Let us now turn to the second example illustrating the analytic potential of Freud's tripartite model of the mind. In the previous section, I remarked that it is not the case that the id always pulls us in one direction, and the superego always in one other direction. I explained this by saying that the id can also pull in different directions simultaneously, and that the same holds true for the superego. There is, however, an even subtler case. *Id and superego can also simultaneously pull in one and the same direction.* This happens when the id forces the superego into its service or, conversely, when the superego forces the id into its service. Let us investigate the former case first.

Take the following examples. An employer criticizes a lazy employee; a schoolteacher upbraids a pupil for truancy; a father smacks his disobedient daughter. Why do they do so? The obvious answer seems to be: because they want to improve the other's behavior; that is, because they want to do good. Looked at in this way, they are driven by their superego. But there is another explanation. They might also do these things because it gives them *sensual pleasure,* a sense of power or sexual excitement. In that case, they are driven by their id. Their id has functionalized their superego. To be sure, they do not criticize, upbraid, and smack for sensual pleasure only. It is more complicated than that. They achieve double satisfaction: the satisfaction that comes from doing the right thing (superego-satisfaction) and the satisfaction that comes from doing the pleasurable thing (id-satisfaction). They are having their cake and eating it.

Such a strategy is not, or at least need not be, conscious. Our fictitious employer, schoolteacher, and father do not feign their desire to do good. Nor is it implied that all people who do good are *really* or *primarily* driven by their id. Freud does not mean to say that we are all conscious cheats or essentially bad, but only that our motivations are a great deal more complex than we tend to think.

Just as intricate as the superego's subjugation by the id is the converse case, in which the id is subjugated by the superego. This happens when people start deriving a kind of perverse pleasure from obeying the superego's demands, pleasure springing not from doing the right thing but from the suffering that so often goes with it. It happens, for example, when a woman with an abusive husband starts deriving a certain satisfaction from her degradation. I am not referring to crude sexual masochism. A masochist welcomes his abuse. A battered woman obviously does not. The satisfaction she achieves — in the case of her id having been subjugated by her superego — is more subtle in nature. Her suffering may make her feel powerful (because she is holding out and not running away); it may make her feel better than her husband (because she has not sunk to his level); it may even make her feel in command (thinking that her suffering is going to win her husband round again). Of course this does not make the physical pain and the mental anguish any less real. It is just that the situation *also* generates pleasurable feelings of power and superiority.

The case, then, is a highly complicated one. The woman's superego impels her to "love, honor, and obey" her husband and thus not to leave him. This produces genuine suffering. Normally, the id would pull her in the opposite direction. But now that her id has been vanquished by her superego, it is no longer able to strive for satisfaction in its own ("selfish," pleasure-oriented) way but only in the ("considerate," sacrifice-oriented) way of the superego. Pleasure can only be achieved through suffering. Superego and id have started to pull in the same direction. It is obvious that this is a psychologically dangerous situation. For such an imbalance between id and superego makes it impossible for the woman's ego to evaluate her relationship realistically. Correspondingly difficult are the problems facing anyone who wants to convince her that she should leave her husband.

For the third illustration of the analytic potential of Freud's tripartite model of the mind we can use the example we have just examined. It not only shows that Freud's model can help to clarify highly complex mental processes. It also illustrates the model's sensitivity to the social and historical embeddedness of these processes. The problem of the woman in our example is not analyzed simply as a conflict between duty and desire, but as resulting from, first, her internalization of problematic social norms and values and, second, the overly strong nature of her superego (that is, of these social norms and values once internalized). Her problem would have been different if she had had the chance to internalize different social norms and values — say, if the social environment in which she grew up had fostered the need to be autonomous instead of the need to "love, honor, and obey." Her problem would also have been different if her education and upbringing had given her a better chance to develop stronger ego and id-processes. (Here, again, it becomes clear that the difference between superego and id is not equivalent to the difference between good and bad. That is why, in the preceding paragraph, I enclosed the words *selfish* and *considerate* in quotation marks.)

Additionally, the woman's problem is affected by her *current* social circumstances. If, for instance, she is financially dependent on her husband, this makes a real difference to her situation, not simply on an "objective" level but also in her conscious and unconscious perception of the problem. The prospect of suddenly being destitute might produce worries and fears on the level of her conscious personality, and it might touch upon preoccupations on the level of the id and the superego. Here, too, we see that the workings of the id, ego, and superego are inextricably linked to the social setting in which they take place and that, conversely, the relevance of this social setting to a person's life cannot be isolated from the workings of his id, ego, and superego. Far from being a mere psycho-logy, a mere science of the psyche, Freudian theory enables us to analyze the *interaction of mental and social processes.*

The Id and Society

There is one thing that, according to Freud, is *not* dependent on social and historical circumstances: the sexual drives of the id. They are the same in all people at all times and all places and cannot be modified. Our superego and ego vary according to time and place (the nineteenth century possessed different social norms and values than does the twenty-first century; America's social norms and values are different from Iran's; a spoiled child will develop a weaker ego than a child that has not been spoiled). Furthermore, the extent to which our id-drives manage to manifest themselves and influence our conscious life is dependent on our ego and superego, hence on education and upbringing, hence on social and historical circumstances; and our worries, fears, traumas, and other preoccupations that we have repressed and that thereby have become part of our id-processes are socially and historically contingent too. *But the original components of the id, the sexual drives with which we are born, are impervious to social and historical change.* These lustful, pleasure-seeking, aggressive, and destructive urges neither alter nor age. They are immutable and immortal.

This state of affairs has important implications for Freud's view of the relationship between the individual and society. It does not make this view any less sophisticated, but it does make it less optimistic. For it implies a fundamental skepticism both towards society as it is and towards society as it might be. It implies that there are in us irredeemably antisocial urges that press blindly and uncompromisingly for satisfaction, irrespective of the consequences. It implies that these urges are to be found even in the noblest of men and women. And it implies that they can never be eradicated. We repress them, satisfy them vicariously through dreams and fantasies, even satisfy them by acting them out — but they can never be satiated and always keep pressing for more. In every man, in every woman, there exists a force that is never content with the satisfactions it achieves and is always at odds with the social demands that society, any society, necessarily places on its members.

This does not mean — the point bears repeating — that the id-drives are bad in themselves. They urge us to seek pleasure and thus provide a necessary counterweight to the superego-drives. Nor does it mean that we are not made to be social, that our true nature is selfish. The id-drives are there before we begin to develop a conscious personality and to internalize social norms and values, but this temporal priority does not entail an ethical priority. We need both id-drives and superego-drives; only when there is a balance between the two can we live happily as social beings. It does mean, however, that deep down in all of us there exists an irreducible antisocial remainder that forever refuses to be socialized. The fit between the individual and society will therefore never be perfect. There will always be the unconscious nagging of the id urging us to transgress. This is what Freud in one of his book titles calls *Das Unbehagen in der Kultur,* man's fundamental unease within civilization.

(The traditional English translation of the title is *Civilization and Its Discontents.*)

Any society is constantly under threat from the antisocial strivings of the id. Our own society is no exception. However civilized and advanced it may appear, indeed however civilized and advanced it may be, our society can never be safe from the drives of the id. The id can break lose at any time. From a Freudian perspective, therefore, any conservative glorification of the status quo is out of the question; not because society is inherently bad but because it contains within itself the seeds of its own destruction.

Just as problematic from a Freudian perspective is the view that glorifies not the present but the future, assuming it to be possible to bring about a truly harmonious society. This view, too, overlooks the fact that the tension between the antisocial drives of the id and the social demands of society can never be overcome. An anecdote in Ernest Jones's biography of Freud illustrates this skeptical psychoanalytic stance rather nicely. Once, Jones relates,

> Freud surprised me by saying he had recently had an interview with an ardent Communist and had been half converted to Bolshevism, as it was then called. He had been informed that the advent of Bolshevism would result in some years of misery and chaos, and that these would be followed by universal peace, prosperity, and happiness. Freud added: "I told him I believed the first half."[8]

Freudian psychoanalysis is not only skeptical about revolutionary utopianism but also about evolutionary utopianism, the belief that political, economic, and technological progress will eventually remove all barriers between people making them (or allowing them to be) truly social beings. To understand this skepticism one needs to look no further than the internet connection provided by the computer on one's desk. A few mouse-clicks and it becomes apparent that even the most modern and socially oriented of technologies cannot escape the pull of the most ancient and antisocial of human drives. Freudian psychoanalysis, then, is incompatible with *any* kind of utopianism, be it of a liberal, neo-liberal, Marxist, neo-Marxist, communist, or any other persuasion.

In this section, I have underlined the ineradicable tension between the id and society. In doing so I may have created the impression that the id and society are simple opposites, warring factions forced to reach a compromise. The situation is, however, more complicated than that. The id and society are not simply opposing forces; they are opposing forces that are peculiarly *entwined*. There is a way in which society is dependent on the id, a way in which society feeds on the id as a parasite feeds on its host. It is not just the case that id-processes sometimes converge with internalized social norms and values, as we observed in the previous section. On a much more fundamental level, id-processes can be seen as the *force behind society*. How can social phenomena result from antisocial drives? What are the ethical implications of this peculiar symbiosis of the id and society? Does it mean that man and society are essentially bad after all? To answer these questions is to explain the very core of Freud's theory. It is to uncover the revolutionary nature of psychoanalysis.

The Revolutionary Nature of Psychoanalysis

Why did psychoanalysis cause a scandal from its very inception? Why was it rejected by the majority of both scholars and laymen?[9] Why was it criticized so vehemently? And why has it remained the object of fierce attacks ever since? These questions are often answered by referring to the subject matter of psychoanalysis. The main obstacle to the scientific and social acceptance of psychoanalysis, it is suggested, lies in its frank discussion of the taboo subject of sexuality. This suggestion is incorrect. Around the turn of the twentieth century there was, particularly in the German-speaking world, a host of writers who openly discussed sexual matters in their works: Iwan Bloch, Magnus Hirschfeld, Richard von Krafft-Ebing, Alfred Blaschko, Oswald Bumke, Enoch Heinrich Kisch, Georg Loewenstein, P. J. Möbius, Siegfried Placzek, Bernhard Stern, Erich Wulffen, and others. Many of them were highly respected psychiatrists, doctors, lawyers, and judges. The psychoanalytic engagement with the subject of sexuality was thus by no means scandalous in itself. Nor was the psychoanalytic interest in "abnormal" forms of sexuality and in sexual disturbances in any way unusual, as a small selection from the literature by the writers mentioned above shows: Krafft-Ebing's *Psychopathia sexualis* (1886), Blaschko's *Syphilis und Prostitution* (1893), Bloch's *Die Prostitution* (1912), Hirschfeld's *Die Homosexualität des Mannes*

(1914) and *Liebesmittel* (Aphrodisiacs, 1930), Placzek's *Das Geschlechts-leben der Hysterischen* (The Sexual Life of Hysterics, 1919), Wulffen's *Das Weib als Sexualverbrecherin* (Female Sex Offenders, 1923) and his *Irrwege des Eros* (Erotic Aberrations, 1929). Indeed, many of these and similar works are considerably more exotic and explicit than Freud's writings. Richard von Krafft-Ebing's *Psychopathia sexualis*, for instance, deals with virtually every imaginable form of sexual behavior and includes detailed case histories of sadomasochism, bestiality, coprophilia, and necrophilia. Yet this book received universal acclaim as a pioneering work of psychiatry; its author, who from 1889 until his retirement in 1902 taught at the same university as Freud, was widely respected throughout his life.

Why, then, is Freud vilified? In what way is his work different from these other publications? Freud does not simply provide new information on sexual matters; *he overhauls the basis upon which they are studied*. He redefines the nature of sexuality and in doing so *transforms our view of what it is to be human*. This radical departure from traditional scholarship has its foundation in three interrelated theses.

First, Freud posits the importance of sexuality (in the extended sense) to *all* aspects of human existence. Sexual gratification is no longer simply seen as one of many things about which people think and to which they aspire; rather, the sexual drive is regarded as constitutive of the way the mind works and thus as affecting all our thoughts and actions. Whereas traditional scholarship removes the threat of sexuality by confining it to one area of life, psychoanalysis does the very opposite.

Second, Freud's approach makes it impossible to view the distinction of normal and abnormal in terms of *us* and *them*. As the book titles above indicate, traditional scholarship considers sadism, masochism, and other forms of sexuality that society condemns to be pathological phenomena, things that *other* people do: perverts, deviants, sex offenders. The psychoanalytic model of sexual development takes away that comfort by making it clear that seemingly pathological urges can be found in all of us. The difference between *us* and *them* is not one between normal people and perverts, but one between potential perverts and actual perverts. Psychoanalysis brings out into the open what is revealed by every war but repressed by every society and every individual: that apparently normal people, too, are subject to lustful, antisocial drives.

Third, Freud conceives of the sexual drive as something that is not, and never will be, under our control. This implies a fundamental skepticism towards the idea of human autonomy. The concept of the id and the superego as unconscious forces involved in all mental processes is fundamentally at odds with the idea that people are in complete control of their destiny. Freud himself describes this implication of psychoanalysis as the *psychological blow to man's vanity;* a third scientific blow for man after the cosmological blow delivered by Copernicus and the biological blow delivered by Darwin.

> In the course of centuries the naïve self-love of men has had to submit to two major blows at the hands of science. The first was when they learnt that our earth was not the centre of the universe but only a tiny fragment of a cosmic system of scarcely imaginable vastness. This is associated in our minds with the name of Copernicus, though something similar had already been asserted by Alexandrian science. The second blow fell when biological research destroyed man's supposedly privileged place in creation and proved his descent from the animal kingdom and his ineradicable animal nature. This revaluation has been accomplished in our own days by Darwin, Wallace and their predecessors, though not without the most violent contemporary opposition. But human megalomania will have suffered its third and most wounding blow from the psychological research of the present time which seeks to prove to the ego that it is not even master in its own house, but must content itself with scanty information of what is going on unconsciously in its mind.[10]

These are the insights, then, that set Freud apart from traditional scholars such as von Krafft-Ebing: no area of life is unaffected by man's sex-drive; no man is free from so-called abnormal sexual tendencies; no man is in complete control of his sex-drive. It is here that the "scandalous" nature of psychoanalysis becomes apparent. For with these insights the usual strategies for dealing with taboo subjects do not work. It is no longer possible to marginalize sexuality by relegating it to an apparently lower sphere of human activity; no longer possible to moralize it away by ascribing the threats it evokes to an evil minority; and no longer possible to defuse it by presenting the shameful things it points to as untypical of human relations. The purity of existence is irretrievably lost. This, then, is what is behind the accusation, made by scholars and laymen alike, that psychoanalysis sexualizes everything, that it is perverted, reductive, one-sided, that it is irrational, illogical, mystical, that it debases man: the revolt against the psychoanalytic destruction of man's image of himself as an essentially rational, self-determined, decent social being.

To be sure, Freud was not the first to question this positive self-image. Many religions stress the sinfulness of human nature; one needs to think only of the Christian doctrine of the Fall of Man. Several philosophers before Freud, too, assumed that there is a strong antisocial streak in man; some of them, such as Friedrich Nietzsche, even referred to unconscious mental processes. But Freud put forward his ideas not as theological dogma or philosophical speculation, but as scientific theory. At the end of the nineteenth century, when theology and philosophy were quickly losing ground to the rising sciences, this empirical approach was bound to have a particularly strong impact. Moreover, in contrast to theological or philosophical positions, Freud offered no religious comfort or redeeming ideology: no prospect of eternal bliss in a hereafter, no Nietzschean vision of a new type of man, no grand proposal offering a way out of the predicament he described. All we can hope to achieve is a little more self-knowledge, a better balance between our contradictory drives. The rest is a matter of muddling through.

But what has all this to do with the workings of society? How do these reflections help us to understand the idea put forward in the previous section that society is dependent on the sexual drives of the id? The answer can be found in the way "normal" people manage to stay "normal"; that is, in the way they manage to redirect their sex-drive from sexual aims to nonsexual ones. In other words, the answer can be found in what in chapter 1 I termed *cultural conversion,* the transformation of antisocial *sexual* impulses into more social *cultural* activities. This conversion thesis can best be explained by contrasting it with two traditional views of the relationship between man and society.

The first of the traditional views sees man as fundamentally good. He may do bad things from time to time, but that is merely the result of ignorance and social circumstance. With sufficient education and in a harmonious social environment his true — good — nature will always assert itself. (With the possible exception of a few misfits who will need to be locked up.) This view does not seem very plausible, and few theorists are prepared to accept it. On the more practical level of everyday discourse, however, it is surprisingly widespread. For example, when children commit crimes, this is often ascribed to the bad influence of the various mass media; without their negative influence, it is implied, a child would not do such things. The view is also implicit in many political discussions. One needs to think only of the common political assumption that racism would disappear if only racists (usually constructed as *them* rather than *us*) knew more about ethnic minorities and lived in different social conditions — an assumption that ignores the likelihood of deep-rooted primitive drives behind racism that awareness training and job creation cannot weed out.

The second traditional view is less simplistic. It assumes that there are good drives *and* bad drives in man; that the good drives push him towards altruistic, social behavior, and the bad drives towards selfish, antisocial behavior; and that, therefore, the stronger his good drives are, the more good actions he will perform. In this view, man's good drives and man's bad drives are clearly distinct qualities pushing him in clearly distinct directions. If the good drives win out, the result is social harmony and peace; if the bad drives win out, the result is crime, social conflict, or war. A better society is a society with better people; the improvement of society a matter of the improvement of man through the elimination of his bad drives. Social progress is human progress.

It will come as no great surprise that Freud does not share the first view. I have, after all, repeatedly pointed out that according to him our lustful, aggressive urges can never be eradicated. But Freud does not share the second view either. According to him, people do not simply have two different original drives, a good one leading to social behavior and a bad one leading to antisocial behavior. At birth, people have only selfish drives; apart from the satisfaction of their nutritive needs, they seek only sensual pleasure, and do so without shame and without regard for the feelings of others. (Earlier I therefore described babies and small children somewhat provocatively as *sex-monsters*.) Growing up, however, they quickly discover that this indiscriminate search for sensual pleasure often has negative consequences: they get punished by their parents, other children no longer want to play with them, and so on. So they start internalizing social norms and values in order to live as social beings. For Freud, then, it is the confrontation with the outside world that leads to the formation of a social conscience, a superego.

This position explodes the second traditional view we looked at in several ways. To begin with, it makes it clear that man's social drives are not simply given, as are his antisocial drives, but are produced by upbringing and education. This means that his social drives do not *naturally* lead to altruistic, social behavior. It is only when and where society praises or condemns certain actions that people are instilled with a desire to carry them out or refrain from them. Moreover, man's social drives can also lead him to destructive, antisocial behavior. For as we saw earlier, people driven predominantly by their superego may well become so critical of the things they see around them that they end up as terrorists. But there is more. As I indicated, the social drives complement the antisocial ones but do not eliminate them. At most they can effect their repression, but even this will take care of man's antisocial dimension only partially. To repress *all* id-drives is impossible (and in any case would be unhealthy). Every man, then, has lustful, aggressive, antisocial drives which he cannot repress and which he must therefore handle differently. His superego will urge him to do this in a socially acceptable way, but how is that possible when the drives are essentially antisocial? He can, of course, act out some wishes, and if he is to stay healthy this is indispensable. Sex with a consenting partner, for example, or the occasional outburst of anger are ways of satisfying his id-drives without endangering the social order. However, the opportunities people have to satisfy their id in this way are limited. So how can the remaining id-pressure be reduced in a socially acceptable manner? Freud's answer is, by transforming lustful, aggressive, antisocial urges into unselfish or even altruistic forms of behavior. People unconsciously *convert* id-energy into cultural activities (in the broadest sense of the word). Instead of beating someone up, they join a boxing club; instead of spying on their attractive next-door neighbor, they read *Playboy;* instead of humiliating people, they become lawyers; instead of turning into perverts, they become sexologists or vice-squad officers; instead of living out their secret urges, they transform them into novels, plays, poems, and paintings. Thus, from a psychoanalytic perspective the second traditional view we looked at above is not only incorrect because man's socially oriented drives do not naturally lead to altruistic, social behavior and may even lead to antisocial behavior, but also because altruistic, social behavior is all too often powered by antisocial drives.

Culture, then, is to a large extent the result of man's unconscious attempts to find nonsexual outlets for sexual drives. Some outlets may betray their origins more clearly than others; reading or writing pornography is more easily identifiable as a desexualized form of sexuality than is reading or writing a poem. Yet they all have the same origin. They all originate in the necessity to satisfy potentially destructive, antisocial urges in a nondestructive, socially sustainable way. In this sense, culture is not so much the grand creation of autonomous individuals as the by-product of an unconscious survival strategy.[11]

From this perspective, even our highest artistic, intellectual, and humanitarian achievements are ultimately expressions of our most primitive urges. A higher, more developed culture therefore does not signify a higher, more developed form of humanity. Culture does not eradicate man's lustful, aggressive urges; it merely provides sophisticated ways of satisfying them in a manner commensurate with the needs and demands of the community. When we now look back for the last time at the second traditional view we examined above, it becomes clear that a better society cannot be a society with better people, but only a society which offers its members better means to absorb their badness. What social progress consists of is not a decrease in antisocial id-drives, but an increase in social id-satisfactions.

The account of Freud's position I have just given may be open to misunderstanding. Let me therefore reiterate two vital points I made earlier. First, Freud does not say that cultural achievements are powered *only* by id-energy. He does not say that when we join a boxing club, become lawyers, or write a poem, we are driven *only* by lustful, aggressive urges. According to him, all these activities are overdetermined, motivated by several wishes at the same time. Thus, someone may want to become a vice-squad officer because (unconsciously) he is fascinated by sexual crimes *and* because (semiconsciously) he wants to have the status that goes with being a policeman *and* because (consciously) he wants to follow in the footsteps of his father, likes the dynamic nature of the job, and is attracted to the working atmosphere within the police force. Of course, conscious and semiconscious wishes may in turn be motivated by wishes of which one is not conscious. A conscious wish to take up the same profession as one's father may well be motivated by the unconscious desire to compete with and outdo him. But conscious and unconscious wishes may also be contradictory. For example, it is entirely possible that someone is unconsciously drawn to sex crimes whilst consciously abhorring them, and that both urges impel him to become a vice-squad officer. But whatever the relationship between the various wishes, they all need to be taken into account when we try to understand the things people do. The id-drives can neither be made the sole explanation of human behavior nor can they be left out of the equation. The former would be reductive, the latter intellectually dishonest.

Second, the fact that even our highest artistic, intellectual, and humanitarian actions are to a greater or lesser extent motivated by sexual impulses does not mean that these actions no longer have any moral content or that we are all entirely evil. It *is* better to be a vice-squad officer than a sex-killer, better to join a boxing club than to beat up one's neighbor, regardless of whether or not there are also less social motives behind these actions. Also, however antisocial some of our urges may be, we *do* possess social urges too. These may not yet exist when we are born, and may be "merely" the result of upbringing and education, but that does not make them any less important.

Freud's position, then, is neither reductive nor nihilistic; it does not reduce humans to id-animals, nor does it erase the difference between good and evil. It does, however, place all our actions under the uncomfortable suspicion that they are not what we think they are. What is more, it places them under the even more uncomfortable suspicion that they may well be the very opposite of what we think they are, that they are what we do not want them to be or what we think they ought not to be. From a psychoanalytic perspective, *nothing* can be taken for granted. The most trivial slips of the tongue can be evidence of the deepest ambivalences; the most common cases of forgetting can be indications of the most painful traumas; the sweetest dreams can hide the nastiest secrets; the highest forms of art can be expressions of the lowest desires; and the most altruistic feelings can have their origins in the most selfish drives.

By seeking out the selfish in the altruistic, the low in the high, the ambivalent in the straightforward, the abnormal in the normal, Freud explodes the binary classifications and clear-cut demarcations that structure our world-view. We like to view ourselves and the world around us in terms of unified entities such as *the mind*, oppositions such as *us/them*, and a host of unambiguous moral principles such as *one should always listen to one's conscience*. Such is the power of this perspective that we remain caught up in it even when we believe we are at our most critical. Thus, we critically observe that we have mixed feelings about something or that we are torn between different desires — but we still view such mental ambiguities as processes from which we can step back, which we can objectify and which are under our control. We condemn abuse of power, racism, and sexual harassment — but we find it impossible to see ourselves as potential fascists, racists, or rapists. We reproach ourselves for not always doing what our conscience tells us to do — but we do not doubt that obeying our conscience is a good thing. *Freud questions all these other things too.*

It is this that constitutes the revolutionary nature of psychoanalysis. Psychoanalysis does not simply provide additional information on, and new ways to deal with, mental ambiguities, sexual problems, deviant behavior, and the like. It transforms the safe framework within which we would like to study these phenomena. In doing so it transforms our view of ourselves and of our relationship with others. Psychoanalysis shows us what we are by confronting us with what we do not want to know.

Notes

[1] This is not to say that before the 1920s Freud did not address this difficulty but only that he did not yet have a fully worked-out theory.

[2] As far as terminology is concerned, Freud's main source was Georg Groddeck's *Das Buch vom Es* (The Book of the It, 1923). Freud himself claimed that Groddeck had borrowed the term from Nietzsche and that his own use of it was influenced by both Groddeck *and* Nietzsche. As Bernd Nitzschke has pointed out, there are some reasons to doubt this. Nietzsche does not use the term *das Es;* and when he uses *es* as a noun, he does so in a critical way. Thus Nietzsche writes in aphorism 17 of *Jenseits von Gut und Böse* (Beyond Good and Evil, 1886) that "it is a *falsification* of the facts to say: the subject 'I' is a condition of the predicate 'think.' It thinks; but that this 'it' is precisely the famous old 'I' is, to put it mildly, only a supposition, an assertion, and definitely not an 'immediate certainty.' Ultimately, even saying 'it thinks' is saying too much: this 'it' already contains an *interpretation* of the process and does not belong to the process itself. . . . [P]erhaps one day even logicians will learn to do without this little 'it' (which is all that is left of the good old I)." According to Nitzschke, Eduard von Hartmann's *Philosophie des Unbewußten* (Philosophy of the Unconscious, 1869) is the more likely precursor. See Bernd Nitzschke,

Aufbruch nach Inner-Afrika. Essays über Sigmund Freud und die Wurzeln der Psycho-analyse (Göttingen: Vandenhoeck & Ruprecht, 1998), 109–74; the quotation from Nietzsche can be found on p. 143. However, as Nitzschke admits, in the eighteenth and nineteenth centuries there were also other writers who contrasted "I" with "it," and influence does not require intellectual agreement. Hence Groddeck's and Freud's source of inspiration does not have to have been von Hartmann and may, in fact, have been Nietzsche after all.

[3] Sigmund Freud, *On Metapsychology,* trans. James Strachey, ed. Angela Richards, vol. 11 of *The Penguin Freud Library,* ed. Angela Richards and Albert Dickson (Harmondsworth: Penguin, 1991), 393.

[4] Freud, *On Metapsychology,* 397.

[5] Calvin S. Hall, *A Primer of Freudian Psychology* (New York: Mentor/New American Library, 1954), 85.

[6] Sigmund Freud, *Civilization, Society and Religion,* trans. James Strachey, ed. Albert Dickson, vol. 12 of *The Penguin Freud Library,* ed. Angela Richards and Albert Dickson (Harmondsworth: Penguin, 1991), 233.

[7] Freud, *Civilization, Society and Religion,* 43.

[8] Ernest Jones, *The Last Phase, 1919–1939,* vol. 3 of Sigmund *Freud: Life and Work* (London: The Hogarth Press, 1957), 17.

[9] To be sure, the scholarly criticism of psychoanalysis was never as unanimous and indiscriminate as Freud believed (or liked to suggest).

[10] Sigmund Freud, *Introductory Lectures on Psychoanalysis,* trans. James Strachey, ed. James Strachey and Angela Richards, vol. 1 of *The Penguin Freud Library,* ed. Angela Richards and Albert Dickson (Harmondsworth: Penguin, 1991), 326.

[11] See Hans-Martin Lohmann, *Freud zur Einführung,* Zur Einführung 71 (Hamburg: Junius, 1986), 37–38.

Part Two:

Literature and Culture

4: The Psychoanalysis of Literature

HOW CAN FREUD'S IDEAS be applied to the study of literature? And how do they contribute to our understanding of the world we live in? These questions are the subject of part 2. I shall be seeking to answer them in as concrete a manner as possible, not through theoretical reflection but by looking at a number of representative psychoanalytic studies of literary and cultural phenomena. The present chapter is devoted to four interpretations of works of fiction: Shakespeare's *Hamlet;* Heine's "Lore-Ley"; and two fairy tales, "The Fisherman and the Jinny," and "Snow White." The next chapter focuses on the psychoanalysis of culture. After a detailed analysis of Freud's *Totem und Tabu,* it examines the way Germany deals with its National Socialist past; the German student revolution of the late 1960s; man's cultural self-deception; and the case of the Belgian pedophile Marc Dutroux and the public reactions to it.

The Mystery of *Hamlet*

It was Freud himself who, through a number of reflections on the play in *Die Traumdeutung,* laid the foundations for the psychoanalytic interpretation of *Hamlet.* These reflections were then amplified by Freud's pupil and biographer Ernest Jones, first in a paper published in 1910 and later in a book entitled *Hamlet and Oedipus* (1949). Before we look at this book in more detail, let us recall the unfolding of events in *Hamlet.*

The play is set in medieval Denmark. Hamlet's father, the king, has just been killed by his brother Claudius, Hamlet's uncle. Claudius has married his brother's wife, Gertrude, and ascended the throne. Hamlet does not know that his father was murdered, but he is extremely upset by his father's death and above all by his mother's marriage to Claudius. A further cause of distress appears to be his lack of success in wooing Ophelia, who is warned by both her father Polonius (the Lord Chamberlain) and her brother Laertes not to trust his advances. Then, his father's ghost appears to him, telling him of the murder and urging him to revenge the crime.

In order to conceal his intentions Hamlet starts behaving as if he were mad, but at the same time devises a plan to ascertain whether Claudius is indeed guilty. He asks a group of actors to perform a play about a man who kills his royal brother and marries the Queen. He will then watch Claudius, and if his uncle flinches, "I know my course" (2.2.94).[1] The play is performed, and Claudius gives himself away. Hamlet now knows that it is incumbent upon him to kill his uncle. The first time he sees him again, however, Claudius is praying, and Hamlet does not want to send him to his death like this because a Claudius killed during "the purging of his soul" would go "to heaven" (3.3.85, 78). Instead, Hamlet goes to his mother, and starts reproaching her for having married Claudius. Suddenly, he realizes that someone is hiding behind the arras and thrusts his rapier right through, killing the person behind it, who turns out to be Polonius.

Claudius, by now seriously worried about Hamlet's behavior, sends his nephew, together with two courtiers (Rosencrantz and Guildenstern), to England in order to have this apparent madman put to death there. But Hamlet finds out about the scheme and, managing to have Rosencrantz and Guildenstern killed instead, returns to Denmark. Upon arrival, he discovers that Ophelia has committed suicide.

Claudius immediately concocts a new plan to get rid of Hamlet. Laertes (Polonius's son and Ophelia's brother) is mad with rage at Hamlet, and Claudius arranges a show duel between Laertes and Hamlet — with the former's rapier dipped in lethal poison. On top of that, Claudius arranges for a poisoned chalice to be offered to Hamlet during the fight. The duel takes place, but it is the Queen who ends up drinking from the chalice. Laertes wounds Hamlet with the poisoned rapier; but when Laertes is forced to drop the weapon, Hamlet grabs it and wounds Laertes. The dying Queen, realizing that the chalice from which she drank contained venom, tells Hamlet that she has been poisoned, whereupon Hamlet kills Claudius. The Queen, Claudius, Laertes, and Hamlet — all are now dead. The play ends with the arrival on the scene of Fortinbras, King of Norway, and his troops. The Norwegian invasion, which had been looming on the horizon from act 1, has become reality.

There are three reasons why Jones (and, before him, Freud) is so interested in this particular play.[2] First, *Hamlet* is generally considered to be one of Shakespeare's most important dramas; insights into it will therefore also provide clues to the workings of the great poet's mind. Second, *Hamlet's* enduring popularity means that it also strikes a chord with us, the readers, so that finding out more about the play may help us to find out more about ourselves. I shall return to these reasons later on. The third reason, which I am concerned with now, is the challenge the play presents to the critics and indeed to anyone who wishes to understand it. *Hamlet* contains a mystery, says Jones, that no one has been able to solve: why is Hamlet so hesitant in avenging his father's death? To this mystery Jones wants to find the key.

According to Jones, there can be little doubt that Hamlet is positively tardy in killing his uncle. He jumps at every opportunity that allows him to postpone the act of revenge. He questions the veracity of the ghost's words, tells himself that he is not up to the job, feels his best opportunity (when Claudius is praying) to be inappropriate, and engages in a useless and dangerous fencing match with someone he knows wants to kill him. Why the delay, why the vacillation? To answer this question Jones first disposes of two rival views, that Hamlet is not capable of decisive action and that there are external circumstances preventing him from carrying out his task.

The first view sees Hamlet either as a weakling, an oversensitive, gentle soul, or as the overreflective intellectual, helpless in the face of the real world. This is unconvincing, says Jones. Hamlet is capable both of vigorous, even impulsive action (as when he kills Polonius) and of carefully planned, cunning action (as when he organizes the play to test his uncle or when he sends Rosencrantz and Guildenstern to their deaths). The second view maintains that Hamlet's task is simply too difficult, suggesting that he not merely has to kill his uncle but bring him to justice in a legal sense. This too is unconvincing according to Jones, if only because a Hamlet faced merely with such external difficulties would have talked about them to his friends or at least referred to them throughout the play, which he does not. Jones therefore concludes that there must be something in the task that is repulsive to Hamlet; something, moreover, of which Hamlet is unaware. For the reasons that Hamlet himself gives for his passivity — that he is too cowardly, that the ghost may not have told the truth, that the time is not right, and so on — are too numerous and contradictory to be credible. Taken separately they may possess a certain plausibility, but "when a man gives at different times a different reason for his conduct it is safe to infer that, whether consciously or not, he is concealing the true reason."[3] And as Hamlet gives these various reasons not to others but to himself, it must be concluded that he is *unconsciously* concealing the true reason. "We can therefore safely dismiss all the alleged motives that Hamlet propounds, as being more or less successful attempts on his part to blind himself with self-deception."[4]

Hamlet, then, is struggling with an inner conflict, a conflict of which he is only vaguely aware. His conscious mind wills him to avenge his father's death; his unconscious mind holds him back, effecting hesitancy and procrastination by calling up various arguments (rationalizations) for inactivity. Here the first outlines of Jones's psychoanalytic approach become visible. Rejecting the "view of man's mind, usually implicit and frequently explicit in psychological writings and elsewhere, [which] regards it as an interplay of various processes that are for the most part known to the subject, or are at all events accessible to careful introspection on his part," Jones assumes instead "that a far greater number of these processes than is commonly surmised arises from origins that he never even suspects." We must see man, he says,

> not as the smooth, self-acting agent he pretends to be, but as he really is, a creature only dimly conscious of the various influences that mould his thought and action, and blindly resisting with all the means at his command the forces that are making for a higher and fuller consciousness.[5]

For Jones, as for Freud, man is not master in his own house.

What are the unconscious forces at work in Hamlet? What precisely is he struggling with? The first thing that strikes the reader, says Jones, is the incommensurate impact on Hamlet of his mother's remarrying compared to his father's death. Hamlet is upset by his father's death, but completely thrown off balance by his mother's marriage to Claudius. Indeed, he is so depressed by what Gertrude has done that he even contemplates suicide.

O that this too too sullied flesh would melt,
Thaw and resolve itself into a dew,
Or that the Everlasting had not fix'd
His canon 'gainst self-slaughter. O God! God!
How weary, stale, flat, and unprofitable
Seem to me all the uses of this world!
Fie on't, ah fie, 'tis an unweeded garden
That grows to seed; things rank and gross in nature
Possess it merely. That it should come to this!
But two months dead — nay, not so much, not two —
So excellent a king, that was to this
Hyperion to a satyr, so loving to my mother
That he might not beteem the winds of heaven
Visit her face too roughly. Heaven and earth,
Must I remember? Why, she would hang on him
As if increase of appetite had grown
By what it fed on; and yet within a month —
Let me not think on't — Frailty, thy name is woman —
A little month, or ere those shoes were old
With which she follow'd my poor father's body,
Like Niobe, all tears — why, she —
O God, a beast that wants discourse of reason
Would have mourn'd longer — married with my uncle,
My father's brother — but no more like my father
Than I to Hercules. Within a month,
Ere yet the salt of most unrighteous tears
Had left the flushing in her galled eyes,
She married — O most wicked speed! To post
With such dexterity to incestuous sheets!

(1.2.129–57)

Now why is Hamlet so disturbed at his mother's behavior? Speedy second marriages are not unusual and do not normally produce this kind of emotional turmoil. The reason cannot merely be that Hamlet dislikes Claudius; his reaction is far too strong for that.[6] Nor can it simply be that Hamlet is disappointed that Claudius robs him of his mother's attention. For that, too, his reaction is too strong and in any case Claudius deprives him of no bigger share in his mother's attention than his father did. Jones therefore surmises that there is a special bond between Hamlet and his mother; that, in fact, Hamlet as a child hated sharing his mother even with his father, that he saw his father as a rival and wanted him out of the way. It is safe to assume, Jones continues, that under the influence of upbringing and education Hamlet repressed such unfilial, antisocial thoughts. Now however, with his early wishes having been fulfilled and yet at the same time thwarted again — his father *is* out of the way and replaced by another family member, but not by Hamlet himself — his repressed childhood desires and frustrations are welling up again. Hamlet, in short, is experiencing the reawakening of his Oedipus complex.

Hamlet and Oedipus

The Oedipus complex is probably Freud's best-known concept. It is also the *most maligned* concept in psychoanalysis. The idea that all boys secretly desire their mothers (and girls their fathers), that the bond between children and parents is to no small extent *sexual* in nature is abhorrent to most people. As a result, it is all too often rejected as simply untrue or as a "kinky" idiosyncrasy attributable to Freud's peculiar family circumstances, his mother having been twenty years younger than his father and younger even than his oldest half-brother. Yet on closer examination the concept makes more sense than at first appears.

As we saw in part 1, for Freud sexuality is not necessarily related to reproduction or even to genitality. It will be remembered that he uses the phrases *sexual* and *sexuality* to include every kind of sensual pleasure. Freud therefore does not imply that children secretly long for sexual intercourse with their parents. What he says is that babies and children naturally focus their attempts to obtain pleasure from the outside world first of all on those who are nearest and closest. That is, the favorite object of the child's pleasure-seeking activities are, after its own body, its parents and especially its mother. In this sense, every child's first love is its mother.[7] Examples of the way the child obtains pleasure through its own body are thumb-sucking and masturbation; examples of the way it obtains pleasure through its parents are sucking at the mother's breast, being rocked in its parents' arms, being rubbed dry after bathing, or playing *horsy-horsy*.

This situation, Freud argues, is bound to lead to competition, competition between son and father (both desiring the mother's affection) and between daughter and mother (both desiring the father's affection). In this competitive situation the parents will usually be relatively secure, having each other's affection in the fullest sense possible. (Which is not to say that the special bond between mother and son is always easy to the father, or that between father and daughter always easy to the mother.) For children the situation is different. They feel much more vulnerable; the boy quickly starts perceiving the father as a rival, and the girl — after having transferred her initial orientation towards the mother onto the father — will start regarding the mother in this way. Each will vie with the rival parent for the affection of the other parent; a process which is perhaps most visible during adolescence. To quote from David Stafford-Clark's persuasive account of this element of Freud's theory:

> the adolescent boy becomes rebellious and challenging to parental authority, often particularly to that of his father, while treating his mother with what often seems to be an uneasy mixture of private affection and public assertion, oscillating between dependence and an attempt to dominate. He shows this by leaving her more things to wash, expecting her to do more for him and, at the same time, refusing to recognize the responsibilities of a grown man in the family in terms of the father's leadership and organization. A girl at the same age will defy her mother but openly seek to win over her father by flagrant displays of feminine attraction, about which she can at first seem naïve and shameless, but which later reveal themselves as experimental trials of her femininity for its final aim in seeking a mate outside the family.[8]

Children not only try to "seduce" the parent whose affections they desire most, they also develop negative feelings towards the rival parent. Such hostility, according to Freud, is particularly pronounced in very young children, who tend to wish their rivals out of the way, dead (in their eyes both amount to the same thing; not yet able to understand the full implications of dying, they interpret *dead* simply as meaning "no longer there"). That is why Freud describes this mental state as the child's Oedipus complex, after the protagonist of Sophocles' play *Oedipus Rex* (425 B.C.), who killed his father and married his mother. This desire to get one parent out of the way in order to have exclusive possession of the other is, of course, highly antisocial and is repressed before the child reaches maturity.[9] Still, the Oedipus complex is a necessary phase for children to go through. As the quotation from Stafford-Clark above indicates, the Oedipal situation and its eventual overcoming constitute a trial period preparing children for the need to find a partner outside the family. As Jones puts it, a "child has to learn how to love just as it has to learn how to walk."[10]

The Oedipus complex is a useful phase, but it is not always overcome successfully. Sometimes a boy remains abnormally attached to his mother, or he maintains a lifelong rivalry with his father. There is also the possibility that Oedipal feelings that have seemingly been overcome resurface later in life, usually as the result of the death of a parent or a similar traumatic experience. *This, according to Jones, is Hamlet's situation.* His father's death and his mother's marriage to his uncle have stirred up his repressed Oedipus complex, generating a conflict between his conscious social wishes and his unconscious antisocial, Oedipal wishes; a conflict of which Hamlet is only vaguely aware, but which determines all his actions.

Jones finds evidence of this not only in Hamlet's hesitancy in revenging his father (which I shall examine in detail in the next section) but also in his relationship with Ophelia. As Jones sees it, Hamlet's attitude towards Ophelia is riven by ambivalence, expressing as it does both a desire to get away from his mother and a desire to get closer to her. On the one hand, Ophelia's modesty and chastity are in sharp contrast to the Queen's sensual nature. It would seem therefore that Hamlet is trying to win the love of a woman who least reminds him of his mother. This psychological process is known as *Reaktionsbildung,* reaction-formation: the attempt to repress a desire by pursuing its opposite. (An example of this on a more conscious level would be the effort to avoid an explosion of anger by being overly polite.) On the other hand, Hamlet also seems to court Ophelia in order to make his mother jealous. This is evident most clearly from the scene preceding the play-in-the-play. Here, Hamlet first refuses his mother's request to sit next to her, sitting down at Ophelia's feet instead ("No, good mother, here's metal more attractive") and then, right in front of his mother, proceeds to tease Ophelia with blatant *double entendres.*

HAM. Lady, shall I lie in your lap?

OPH. No, my lord.

HAM. I mean, my head upon your lap.

OPH. Ay, my lord.

HAM. Do you think I meant country matters?[11]

OPH. I think nothing, my lord.

HAM. That's a fair thought to lie between maids' legs.

(3.2.110–17)

Hamlet's Inner Conflict

Let us return to the key issue of the play, Hamlet's procrastination. The psychoanalytic insights considered above allow Jones to explain *why* exactly Hamlet is so tardy in killing his uncle. It is obvious that the reason cannot simply be that Hamlet "secretly wants to sleep with his mother," as the popular vulgarization of Jones's view would have it. If this had been Hamlet's main motivation, he would have got rid of his uncle in no time. The reason is, on the contrary, that Hamlet's flared-up passion for his mother — his Oedipus complex — is not his main motivation; that it is in fact only one forceful motivation among other, equally forceful, motivations; and that moreover these various motivations push him in different directions. Hamlet is suffering from an inner conflict between contradictory impulses.

The precise nature of this conflict becomes clear when we look once again at Claudius's crime. Claudius has killed the king and married the queen. This has two consequences. For one thing, Claudius has now become Hamlet's (second) father; for another, it is now incumbent upon Hamlet to revenge his (first) father. What inner conflict does this produce according to Jones?

First, every time Hamlet starts thinking about his uncle's crime he touches upon his own repressed wishes. For Claudius has done the two very things Hamlet himself unconsciously wanted to do. To reflect on his uncle's crime, on the need for revenge, on possible ways to carry out this revenge — all this is tantamount to reactivating thoughts whose existence Hamlet does not want to acknowledge. "He is therefore in a dilemma between on the one hand allowing his natural detestation of his uncle to have free play, a consummation which would stir still further his own horrible wishes, and on the other hand ignoring the imperative call for the vengeance that his obvious duty demands."[12]

Second, by condemning his uncle, Hamlet would in effect condemn himself. That is, to accept the ethical proposition that Claudius must die would be to accept that he, Hamlet, must die too. The moral fates of Hamlet and Claudius are inextricably linked.

Third, killing his uncle would be equivalent to killing his father, for it is now Claudius who is married to the queen. This again adds to the dilemma. Committing this ultimate sin is something that Hamlet both desires and, under the influence of upbringing and education, abhors.

Fourth and last, Hamlet is torn by the dimly conscious knowledge that by killing Claudius he would not only be revenging his father but also paving the way for his own possession of his mother. It is not a coincidence when Hamlet, without realizing the full meaning of his own words, says that he is driven to revenge "by heaven and hell" (2.2.580). In this sense, to kill Claudius would be to honor his father's memory and besmirch it at the same time.

Add to all this the subsidiary motivation that by doing away with his uncle Hamlet would remove the one obstacle standing between him and the throne, and the full ambivalence of his state of mind becomes apparent. *It is this ambivalence, says Jones, that makes Hamlet procrastinate;* it paralyzes all action "at its very inception."[13]

As Jones makes clear, Hamlet's inner conflict determines not only his action (or rather non-action) towards Claudius, but also towards the other characters in the play. For with their direct outlet blocked, Hamlet's pent-up emotions have to find vent in other directions. This explains his wild and contradictory reproaches of Ophelia, who is accused both of being too prudish (that is, of not being enough like his mother) and of being too lustful (that is, of being too much like his mother). The most succinct expression of this split can be found in Hamlet's sarcastic advice "Get thee to a nunnery" (3.1.121), "for in Elizabethan, and indeed in later, times this was also a term for a brothel; the name 'Covent Garden' will elucidate the point to any student of the history of London."[14] Hamlet's constant harassment of Polonius can be explained along similar lines. Exhibiting the very traits children dislike most about their parents (meddling, prying, and preaching) the Lord Chamberlain offers Hamlet an ideal opportunity to displace, and thus to some extent reduce, his hostility towards Claudius. And it is precisely because Polonius functions as a kind of substitute-Claudius to Hamlet and yet is not his actual father that Hamlet remains so strangely without remorse after stabbing him. Hamlet's own justification — that he mistook Polonius for Claudius — makes no objective sense; after all, Hamlet has just seen Claudius praying in another part of the castle. What Hamlet says makes sense only psychologically, as an indication of the extent to which his uncle and Polonius are identified in his mind. Last but not least, Hamlet's attitude to his mother is also determined by his ambivalent state of mind. Unconsciously enamored with her but unable to express his desire directly, he is forced into giving vent to it indirectly. Thus, he unconsciously attempts to make his mother jealous by flirting with Ophelia, and he bitterly condemns her marriage to Claudius and her wantonness — as he sees it — towards her new husband. These condemnations are particularly telling.

> Nay, but to live
> In the rank sweat of an enseamed bed,
> Stew'd in corruption, honeying and making love
> Over the nasty sty!
>
> (3.4.91–94)

The picture here is one of Gertrude wallowing in her bed that is *enseamed* (greasy with her secretions and Claudius's semen), hot and sweaty (*stew'd* also suggesting "stew," brothel) from sexual intercourse. And when Gertrude asks him what she should do, he answers:

> Not this, by no means, that I bid you do:
> Let the bloat King tempt you again to bed,
> Pinch wanton on your cheek, call you his mouse,
> And let him, for a pair of reechy kisses,
> Or paddling in your neck with his damn'd fingers,
> Make you to ravel all this matter out
> That I essentially am not in madness,
> But mad in craft.
>
> (3.4.182–90)

On the surface, Hamlet's condemnation of his mother's incestuous behavior indicates nothing but disgust, but his laboring the point in graphic detail betrays his fascination. Consciously meaning to say one thing, he unconsciously expresses another; his words are dripping with repressed sexual desire.

How is Hamlet's inner conflict resolved? How does he finally manage to kill his uncle? The answer is straightforward enough. Hamlet does not actually overcome his ambivalence; he never even really attempts to penetrate the darkness of his unconscious. It is only after external circumstances have removed some of the main elements of his dilemma that he is able to act. Only when he and Gertrude are dying, and when he knows that they are dying, is he able to avenge his father's death. Killing Claudius now no longer has anything to do with Hamlet wanting to have his mother all to himself, and any worries about the link between his own moral fate and that of his uncle have become irrelevant. Now, his unconscious no longer holds him back, or at least not enough to prevent him from doing his duty — and he stabs Claudius with the same poisoned rapier that he knows has been his own undoing.

The Play, the Author, the Readers

Psychoanalytic literary criticism is not simply about interpreting a text's protagonists. It also seeks to relate the text to the mind of its author. Everything people do depends on their mental states — on conscious deliberations, conflicts, and decisions, but also on unconscious mental processes — and can therefore be interpreted in psychoanalytic terms. This holds true for the writing of literary texts as well. Indeed, the creative process is among the psychoanalyst's favorite objects of research, because the unconscious element in it is particularly strong. Like dreaming, the creative process provides a valve to the pressure of the unconscious. The creation of literary fictions allows the writer to work his repressed desires out of his system by expressing them in a cloaked, socially acceptable form (without being aware that this is what he is doing). To take up a term I introduced in part 1, *Hamlet* and other works of art are manifestations of *sublimation,* the redirection of sexual energy into higher cultural activities. Thus, just as the interpretation of dreams provides insights into the mind of the dreamer, so the interpretation of literary texts provides insights into the mind of the author. Conversely — and this too is similar to the process of interpreting dreams — insights into the mind of the author provide important clues to the meaning of the text. From a psychoanalytic point of view, text and author are intimately linked.

Psychoanalytic literary criticism does not confine its attention to the relationship between text and author. It also takes account of a third element, the reader. Readers react to what they read in a variety of ways; they like it, love it, admire it, loathe it, are abhorred or fascinated by it, and so on. These feelings reveal a great deal about those who have them, but they may also point to specific themes, motifs, structures *in the text,* to features of the text that an emotionally uninvolved interpretation might miss. Paying attention to such emotional responses can therefore be a great help in uncovering textual phenomena relevant to the understanding of literary texts. Such an approach does not in any way imply a lack of methodological rigor. Like psychoanalysis, psychoanalytic literary criticism is a rational activity; it is not founded on readers' responses but merely seeks to use them as an additional source of information. Of course, the inclusion of readers' responses is not always possible or practicable, and many psychoanalytic interpretations have to manage without them (and often do so quite well). Still, the analysis of the way people respond to literary texts remains a valuable tool of the psychoanalytically oriented critic.

What are the implications of all this for *Hamlet,* the text we are concerned with here? How does Jones relate the text to its author and its readers? To start with the author, the first thing that Jones points to is the hidden nature of Hamlet's conflict. Why, he asks, does the play contain only vague hints and no clear indication as to the cause of Hamlet's procrastination? His answer is that Shakespeare was unable to show the conflict in a clear light because he himself "was unaware of its nature."[15] The play is the guise in which Shakespeare's repressed emotions find expression in a way that Shakespeare himself is not aware of and is not able to control. These emotions, Jones maintains, are Oedipal in nature: Hamlet's Oedipal conflict is "an echo of a similar one in Shakespeare himself."[16] This explains well why the reasons for Hamlet's procrastination are so unclear and why the play remained a mystery for so long.

Of course, this theory is difficult to substantiate; not simply because Shakespeare is no longer around but because we have very little biographical information on him. There are no letters, no diaries, no autobiography — the kind of sources that allow us to speculate with a fair degree of confidence about the mental states of a writer. There are, however, two significant historical facts we do have. We know that Shakespeare's father died in 1601; and we know that *Hamlet* was officially registered at Stationers' Hall (that is, entered on a list of copyrighted works) in 1602. The first pirated edition of the play appeared in 1603, the first official edition in 1604–5. It is therefore reasonable to assume that Shakespeare wrote *Hamlet* under the influence of his father's death; that, indeed, his father's death reawakened repressed desires that then found their way into the play. Additional evidence, Jones says, can be found in some of Shakespeare's other works, particularly in the sonnets with their strong homosexual or bisexual content. The way the *I* of the sonnets is torn between a mature woman (the *dark lady*) and a young man (the *lovely boy*) is an unmistakable indication of an unsuccessfully overcome Oedipal fixation on the mother. That Shakespeare married a woman eight years his senior (a fact not mentioned by Jones) ties in with this.[17]

To avoid misunderstanding, Jones does not say that the play is *merely* a vehicle for Shakespeare's repressed emotions. No work of art, certainly no great work of art, can ever be reduced to its unconscious roots. However strong the writer's unconscious impulses may be, he also creates deliberately, purposefully. Every text is also the product of conscious motivations and as such a carefully organized, highly interlinked unity. To take up again a term introduced in part 1, every work of art is *overdetermined*. Psychoanalytic literary criticism therefore does not uncover *the* meaning of literary texts, but only a specific *layer* of meaning. As Freud puts it:

> all genuinely creative writings are the product of more than a single motive and more than a single impulse in the poet's mind, and are open to more than a single interpretation.[18]

The psychoanalytic interpretation can either contradict other interpretations (as Jones's interpretation contradicts the view of Hamlet as an oversensitive weakling) or complement them. But even if the psychoanalytic reading contradicts existing readings, this does not mean that one is compelled to choose between them. One can also accept both, as an acknowledgment of a fundamental tension in the text. Just as psychoanalysis can reveal contradictory tendencies in someone's decision to become a lawyer or a vice-squad officer (see chapter 3), so psychoanalytic literary criticism can reveal contradictory tendencies in literary texts. This is precisely what most modern psychoanalytic interpretations aim for: not to replace existing interpretations, but to render visible additional layers of meaning that together with the traditionally established meaning or meanings make up the complexity of the text as a whole.

Turning now to the reader (and spectator), we encounter a link similar to the one between *Hamlet* and Shakespeare. The play's popularity, Jones asserts, is founded on the fact that the readers, too, are emotionally involved in the play's central conflict to a high degree. Of course, not all readers suffer from an unsuccessfully overcome Oedipus complex, but they will at least have had their Oedipal phase during childhood. As childhood experiences are central to the person we become, it is not surprising that a play that touches upon our deepest and darkest childhood wishes should hold such a fascination for readers from all times and places. "So we reach the apparent paradox," Jones concludes, "that the hero, the poet, and the audience are all profoundly moved by feelings due to a conflict of the source of which they are unaware."[19]

Of course, it is not merely the topic that has made the play so popular. The last thing Jones wants to do is psychoanalyze away the importance of Shakespeare's genius. All he says is that, besides literary reasons, there are psychological reasons for *Hamlet*'s enduring appeal: the fact that it is rooted in the most basic and most intense unconscious mental struggles humans are faced with.

Psychoanalysis and Literary Criticism

Having examined the psychoanalytic interpretation of *Hamlet,* we must now address the question that logically follows from it: how does this kind of interpretation work with other texts? Is Jones's interpretation not uniquely fitted to *Hamlet* with its strong emphasis on family relations, on filial, paternal, and sexual love? What about texts that deal with totally different topics, that are not about family relations, that do not even include different-sex protagonists?

There are two answers to this. To begin with, psychoanalysis is not, as popular prejudice would have it, concerned merely with "sex" or with "boys being in love with their mothers," but with the much more fundamental problem of the relationship between conscious and unconscious mental processes and the way they determine human behavior. Psychoanalytic tools can therefore be used to examine a whole range of different actions by a whole range of different protagonists. We have already seen this with the theory of faulty actions in part 1, when we looked at passages from Shakespeare's *The Merchant of Venice* and Galsworthy's *The Island Pharisees*. The majority of psychoanalytic theories and concepts — projection, reaction-formation, displacement, sublimation, id/ego/superego, and so on — can be applied in this way. Of course, the characters in a literary text are not actually alive and in that sense they are different from the living human beings psychoanalysis is normally concerned with. But no sensible interpretation of literary texts, at least of realistic literary texts, is possible without the assumption that the characters are people like you and me. That is how the author meant them to be; that is the reason why we are interested in them; that is the basis for our interpretation of their actions and motivations; and that, precisely, is what makes it possible to apply theories and concepts such as projection and reaction-formation to them. As indicated, this argument holds for realistic texts only. Other texts — fairy tales and certain types of poetry are among the most obvious examples — cannot, or can only to a limited degree, be interpreted like this. The only way psychoanalysis can shed light on such forms of fiction is by interpreting them in terms of the psychological function they fulfill for their authors and readers. This brings us to the second answer to the questions posed above.

Psychoanalytic criticism is not restricted to texts with specific themes or specific characters, because *every* literary expression is the result of a complex interaction between the author's conscious and unconscious mental processes and can thus be illuminated by psychoanalytic means. Jones does precisely this when he interprets Hamlet's Oedipal conflict as an unconsciously determined echo of a similar conflict in Shakespeare himself. Admittedly, the situation is usually more complicated than this relatively straightforward example suggests. For in a way creative writing is like dreaming. When people dream, their unconscious wishes (the latent dream-thoughts) are transformed through such mechanisms as displacement, symbolization, and condensation into the manifest dream-content. Instead of dreaming about his mother, a man may dream about his aunt; instead of dreaming about a penis, he may dream about a pen; and when he dreams about hitting his teacher, this may be a condensed image of his aggressive feelings towards his father and towards his brother. According to psychoanalysis, similar transformations take place during the creative process. The writer's unconscious preoccupations find expression in a modified, distorted form rather than simply and directly.

In this sense, *Hamlet* must be considered untypical of the relationship between text and author. Although the play — its location, time, characters, and action — is obviously not simply a copy of its author's mind, the conflict of its main protagonist is still similar to that of the author and has not undergone significant transformation. Yet even this play contains a number of distortions similar to those found in dreams. Jones touches upon this when he discusses the relationship between *Hamlet* and a large group of "Hamletean" legends, including Sophocles' *Oedipus Rex* and the story of Amleth, by Saxo Grammaticus (ca. 1150–1220), which was probably one of the main sources of the play.

> The fundamental theme common to all the members of the group is the success of a young hero in displacing a rival father. In its simplest form the hero is persecuted by a tyrannical father, who has usually been warned of his approaching eclipse, but after marvellously escaping from various dangers he avenges himself, often unwittingly, by slaying the father. . . . In some types of the story the hostility to the father is the predominating theme, in others the affection for the mother, but as a rule both of these are more or less plainly to be traced.[20]

Shakespeare's *Hamlet,* says Jones, is one of many variations of this more general Hamlet myth. For example, the king (old Hamlet) and Claudius can be seen as resulting from the *decomposition* of the original father figure. Decomposition can be understood as inverted condensation; instead of blending different ideas into one, it *disunites* the various components of one idea (or, as in this case, of one person). Thus old Hamlet possesses the more positive, benevolent characteristics of the original father, Claudius the more negative, tyrannical ones. Polonius can be regarded as a third split-off, incorporating the father's didactic character traits. Another process of transformation is the introduction of *subsidiary themes* such as the father-daughter complex and the brother-sister complex exhibited by Polonius and Laertes, who both are conspicuously protective of Ophelia. The third and last dreamwork-like transformation that Jones identifies in the play is the *doubling* of principal characters, the chief motive for which is "the desire to exalt the importance of these [principal characters], and especially to glorify the hero, by decoratively filling in the stage with lay figures of colourless copies whose neutral movements contrast with the vivid activities of the principals."[21] Among the not entirely convincing examples that he gives are Horatio, Marcellus, and Bernardo.

For Jones, all these transformations are transformations of the Hamlet myth, or perhaps it would be better to say of the Oedipus myth. This myth in turn he regards as the expression of childhood wishes common to all human beings, as — to use Carl Gustav Jung's phrase, which Jones borrows in this connection — an expression of the individual's *collective unconscious.* There is, however, another way of treating such transformations. They can also be linked up with the author's *personal unconscious.* That is to say, when confronted with a literary text the psychoanalytic critic is by no means forced to trace it back to a more general myth and thereby to the unconscious preoccupations shared by all humans. Indeed, with many texts there will not even exist such an overarching myth. What the psychoanalytic critic can also do, and what in fact is by far the more common practice, is to identify and interpret transformations as transformations of the author's personal "drama," his mental history. In this way, psychoanalytic criticism can operate without being restricted to texts with a specific set of topics and characters or to texts with a realistic style. To give a few hypothetical examples, an author's repressed homosexuality may be transformed into a story about two repellent women; his doubts about his choice of profession into a story about the competition between an artist and a businessman; and a poem about a withering plant may be expressive of his fear of growing old.

Linking up a text with its author's mental disposition can only be done properly by *inter*linking the two. In the interpretation of dreams, the things the analyst has found out about the dreamer's conscious and unconscious personality are used to understand the dream, and the things he has found out about the dream are used to understand the dreamer's personality. Equally, the psychobiographical interpretation of literary texts is a two-way process: the interpretation of the author and the interpretation of the text go side by side, the one constantly illuminating and modifying the other.

Admittedly, if applied uncritically this type of literary criticism is bound to lead to an overly speculative reading of texts. Moreover, it is always in danger of becoming reductive, of interpreting texts solely in terms of their authors' psychologies — a danger to which Freud himself alerts us, as we saw in the previous section. A more cautious and modest use of psychobiographical criticism, however, can yield genuine insights both into the author's mind and into his oeuvre.

Unconscious Communication:
Heine's "Lore-Ley"

Psychoanalytic criticism, I claimed in the previous section, can be used to interpret the whole range of literary expressions, including poems and fairy tales — texts for which such a reality-based type of interpretation might at first sight seem unsuitable. When applied to such difficult texts, I said, psychoanalytic criticism focuses on the relationship between the text and its author, or between the text and its readers, or both. It elucidates these texts by interpreting them as artistic transformations of the author's mental disposition, or by explaining their enduring appeal on the basis of the psychological fascination they hold for the reader. We gained an impression of how this works when we examined *Hamlet,* but I wish to illustrate this approach more extensively by looking at two analyses of other texts. This section is therefore devoted entirely to Walter Schönau's analysis of "Lore-Ley," by Heinrich Heine (1797–1856), and the next section to Bruno Bettelheim's study of fairy tales.

"Lore-Ley" is one of the best-known poems in German literature. It was written in 1823, first published in 1824, and then included in *Buch der Lieder* (Book of Songs, 1827), Heine's most famous collection of poetry.

Ich weiß nicht, was soll es bedeuten,
Daß ich so traurig bin;
Ein Mährchen aus alten Zeiten,
Das kommt mir nicht aus dem Sinn.

I do not know why it should be,
but I am so sad:
there is an old-time fairy-tale
which I can't put out of my mind.

Die Luft is kühl und es dunkelt,
Und ruhig fließt der Rhein;
Der Gipfel des Berges funkelt
Im Abendsonnenschein.

The air is cool and the twilight is falling
and the Rhine is flowing calmly by;
the top of the mountain is glittering
in the evening sun.

Die schönste Jungfrau sitzet
Dort oben wunderbar,
Ihr goldnes Geschmeide blitzet,
Sie kämmt ihr goldnes Haar.

Up there the most gorgeously beautiful
maiden is sitting;
her golden jewellery sparkles
and she is combing her golden hair.

Sie kämmt es mit goldnem Kamme,
Und singt ein Lied dabey;
Das hat eine wundersame,
Gewaltige Melodey.

She is combing it with a golden comb
and singing a song as she does so;
it has a wonderful
compelling melody.

Den Schiffer, im kleinen Schiffe,
Ergreift es mit wildem Weh;
Er schaut nicht die Felsenriffe,

Er schaut nur hinauf in die Höh'.

It makes a wild nostalgia possess
the boatman in his boat;
he pays no attention to the submerged
     rocks,
he can only look up and up.

Ich glaube, die Wellen verschlingen
Am Ende Schiffer und Kahn;

Und das hat mit ihrem Singen
Die Lore-Ley gethan.

In the end, if I remember rightly,
the waves swallow up the boatman and
     his boat
And that is what she has done,
the Lorelei and her singing.[22]

Walter Schönau's starting-point is the question implicit in the first stanza's "I do not know why it should be, / but I am so sad" and the uncertainty expressed by the last stanza's "if I remember rightly."[23] Here, he points out, Heine diverges the most from such predecessors as Clemens Brentano, who had also written Lore-Ley poems. Whereas they tell the story of the beautiful seductress straight out, Heine's poem includes a subjective framework articulating the author's emotional involvement. His text presents the *Mährchen aus alten Zeiten* as a spontaneous thought — a free association, as it were — prompted by the author's melancholy. As a result, the fatal encounter with the Lore-Ley appears as a kind of mythical model of a similarly devastating experience of the author. That there was indeed such an experience is confirmed, Schönau says, by what we know about Heine's life. Heine research tells us that the poems of *Buch der Lieder* have their psychological roots in Heine's love for his attractive cousin Amalie. Amalie rejected Heine, and it was this traumatic experience that inspired his early poetry and the adaptation of Petrarchism — the poetical treatment of a man's unhappy love for a beautiful woman — that is at the heart of it.[24] From this perspective, "Lore-Ley" is one manifestation of the author's attempt to come to terms, through the medium of literature, with a recent "Liebeskatastrophe," to use Gerhard Höhn's phrase.[25]

However, Schönau says, the poem is much more than that. The story of the Lore-Ley points to a realm that transcends individual experience. It represents a fantasy to be found from ancient Greece to Hollywood: the image of the femme fatale, of woman as an alluring yet dangerous temptress. This image is highly ambivalent, expressing as it does both desire and fear. The occurrence of this universal fantasy suggests that there is more at stake than the unhappy love for Amalie. Through the story of the Lore-Ley, a more basic disappointment becomes visible, that of the child forced to renounce its claim to the mother. Heine's traumatically unsuccessful wooing of Amalie stirred memories of his repressed Oedipal phase — of the child caught between desire and fear of fulfillment, and of the eventual abandonment of its erotic wishes.

This is corroborated, Schönau argues, by the universal popularity of "Lore-Ley." The poem has appealed to people from all times and places because it evokes humanity's principal *Urphantasie*. More than being simply an esthetically pleasing treatment of an interesting topic, it articulates affects which all of us have experienced and were then obliged to repress, but which we re-experience in reading the poem. Of course, neither author nor reader is aware of this. As with *Hamlet*, the communication between them takes place on an unconscious level. This is possible because, as Freud puts it,

> everyone possesses in his unconscious mental activity an apparatus which enables him to interpret other people's reactions, that is, to undo the distortions which other people have [unconsciously] imposed on the expression of their feelings.[26]

Reading amounts to an unconscious decoding of the author's unconscious fantasies. Just as literature allows the author to *express* his repressed affects *in an unconscious, cloaked, and socially acceptable manner,* so it offers the reader the opportunity to *share* in these affects *in the same manner.* From this perspective, the lines "I do not know why it should be, / but I am so sad" are actually true. They are true, first of all, of Heine (even though on a conscious level he may well have used them merely as a literary device). But they are equally true of the reader, who does not understand *his* melancholy fascination.

Like dreams, literature represents a trade-off "between disclosure and concealment."[27] The reader's unconscious is both provoked and pushed back, aroused yet kept at a distance. Reading is a battle between drives and repressions, between the desire for expression and the need for censorship. It engages the mind in its full complexity — as long as the tension between the reader's contradictory impulses is maintained. This, indeed, is the psychoanalytic criterion of esthetic value.

In brief, literary texts do not simply *result* from a conflict between consciousness and unconsciousness but *embody* it. Their artistic greatness, judged by its psychological dimension, depends on the extent to which they allow the reader to re-enact this conflict.

According to Schönau, the psychological tension in "Lore-Ley" is maintained by the fact that the analogy between the poet's and the boatman's fates remains implicit. The poet does not know why he should be so sad, and it is not apparent what the motivating force behind his reminiscence of the Lore-Ley story is. This textual openness, Schönau says, is not only a literary device, employed to enhance the poem's suggestive nature; viewed psychoanalytically, it is also a defense mechanism, a manifestation of the author's unconscious attempt to repress his sexual trauma. On this deeper level, the lines "I do not know why it should be, / but I am so sad" and "if I remember rightly" signify a fundamental ambivalence. They demonstrate that the author feels drawn towards the story of the temptress and her victim *and* is trying not to identify with it. They are both an expression of emotional involvement and a symptom of resistance. For the reader, the subjective framework fulfills a similar function, drawing him in and at the same time foreclosing direct identification. It involves him in the story and turns him into a participant, but the lack of knowledge and the uncertainty it expresses objectify the events again and turn him into a spectator. The reader is caught between desire and repression.

Schönau's interpretation ties in with what we know about Heine's early poetry.[28] The Oedipal constellation identified in "Lore-Ley" is reflected in *Buch der Lieder's* central theme, the union of desire and frustration. Of course, *Buch der Lieder* cannot be reduced to a single concern. It offers social criticism, exposing hypocrisy and deriding petty-bourgeois morality, and addresses philosophical and religious issues. It also represents a critical engagement with conventional Romantic modes of expression, whose inadequacy to the modern world is brought into relief through parody, irony, and deliberate stylistic incongruity.[29] Still, the treatment of the union of desire and frustration clearly stands out. The *I* in the poems continually finds itself trapped "between erotic wishes and bitter forced renunciation, between its irresistible hankering after sexual fulfillment and its incessant pain over the hopelessness of this desire."[30] Again and again, the beloved woman rejects her suitor's advances or turns out to be unavailable. The love in *Buch der Lieder* is therefore distinctly ambivalent in nature, causing as it does both pleasure and pain. How hopeless the situation is can be inferred from two of the book's best-known poems, "Die Lotosblume ängstigt / Sich vor der Sonne Pracht" (The lotus-flower is afraid / of the sun's splendor) and "Ein Fichtenbaum steht einsam" (A fir-tree stands alone). By transposing the book's central theme to the realm of nature, these poems about the impossible love of the lotus-flower and the moon and about the spruce's equally impossible yearning for the palm-tree underscore the inescapability of the frustration. Finally, in this erotic constellation it is the woman who plays the dominant part. The man is passive, dependent, vulnerable — like a son towards his mother. All this lends credence to Schönau's psychoanalytic interpretation of "Lore-Ley."

But there is more. The poems of *Buch der Lieder* seem to act as a kind of self-therapy. By his endless variations on the same erotic theme, Heine appears to make just as many unconscious attempts to get over a sexual trauma. The compulsive way in which he works through all the various aspects of the union of desire and frustration is therefore also to be seen as a psychological working through; it represents "what Freud has termed *Durcharbeiten* [working-through], a process in which an obsessively recurring experience is eventually overcome."[31] The psychological function that Schönau ascribes to "Lore-Ley" is thus confirmed by what we know about *Buch der Lieder* as a whole.

Snow White, or the Meaning and Importance of Fairy Tales

More than any other type of fiction, fairy tales appear at first sight to be resistant to psychoanalytic interpretation. The fantastic events they describe are, it would seem, much too far removed from reality to be accessible to an approach developed through analyses of the real problems of real people. Moreover, the fairy tales we know today are the result of centuries of storytelling. Since they do not have one author, or even a group or collection of identifiable authors, they cannot be explained on the basis of their creator's psychology. But appearances can be deceptive. In fact, psychoanalysis has much to contribute to our understanding of fairy tales, as can be seen from Bruno Bettelheim's classic study *The Uses of Enchantment*, first published in 1976.

The Uses of Enchantment deals with a variety of fairy tales, including those of Sindbad the Sailor and Sindbad the Porter, Hansel and Gretel, Little Red Riding Hood, Jack and the Beanstalk, Cinderella, and Snow White.[32] Bettelheim examines these stories in terms of the function they fulfill for their main audience, the children who read or listen to them. His thesis is that fairy tales help children to overcome the psychological problems inherent in growing up, thus enabling them to develop a well-balanced personality. When examined from this psychoanalytic perspective, fairy tales reveal a wealth of unconscious meanings.

All children, Bettelheim says, are faced with a multitude of problems and challenges. They need to restrain primitive urges, overcome Oedipal and sibling rivalries, learn to respect other people and value social relationships while freeing themselves from immature dependencies, gain individuality and self-esteem, and develop a moral sense. These problems and challenges are extremely vexing for the child, but their true nature usually remains in the dark. Children, particularly young children, do not really understand what they are going through and are unaware, or only dimly aware, of the source of their confusion. And even if they were intellectually capable of comprehending their predicament, they would still lack the emotional security to face up to it. Consequently, they are unable to cope with their plight in the way adults would. To provide children with rational explanations and to encourage them to deal with their difficulties consciously and rationally, as "enlightened" parents tend to do, will therefore only exacerbate their inner turmoil. (Here, Bettelheim remarks ironically that in "trying to get a child to accept scientifically correct explanations, parents all too frequently discount scientific findings of how a child's mind works."[33]) Children need to work on their difficulties in a way they can handle. They need to find a way of confronting their confusion, of making their unconscious wishes and fears conscious, without being overwhelmed. It is here that fairy tales become important.

Fairy tales, Bettelheim asserts, are to be seen as transformations of unconscious material into conscious fantasies. They offer symbolic representations of children's deepest wishes and fears, thereby allowing them to reduce mental tension. Through reading and listening to fairy tales, children externalize their inner conflicts and enact possible solutions. Fairy tales thus function not just on a conscious but also on an unconscious level; they convey both overt and covert meanings. On a conscious level, they are simply good stories that depict fantastic events and entertain the youthful reader or listener in an exciting, romantic, or humorous fashion. On an unconscious level, "these stories speak to his budding ego and encourage its development, while at the same time relieving preconscious and unconscious pressures. As the stories unfold, they give conscious credence and body to id pressures and show ways to satisfy these that are in line with ego and superego requirements."[34] Bettelheim's analysis of the tale of the fisherman and the Jinny may serve as an example.

"The Fisherman and the Jinny" is part of *Thousand and One Nights,* the famous Indian-Persian collection of fairy tales. Its central theme, however, can be found in all cultures. The Brothers Grimm's *Kinder- und Hausmärchen,* for example, contains a similar story, "Der Geist im Glas" (The Spirit in the Bottle).

> "The Fisherman and the Jinny" tells how a poor fisherman casts his net into the sea four times. First he catches a dead jackass, the second time a pitcher full of sand and mud. The third effort gains him less than the preceding ones: potsherds and broken glass. The fourth time around, the fisherman brings up a copper jar. As he opens it, a huge cloud emerges, which materializes into a giant Jinny (genie) that threatens to

kill him, despite all the fisherman's entreaties. The fisherman saves himself with his wits: he taunts the Jinny by doubting aloud that the huge Jinny could ever have fitted into such a small vessel; thus he induces the Jinny to return into the jar to prove it. Then the fisherman quickly caps and seals the jar and throws it back into the ocean.[35]

The first story-element that Bettelheim addresses is the Jinny's desire to kill the fisherman. As the story goes, during the first hundred years of captivity the Jinny intended to make the person rich who would set him free. Then, for four centuries he intended to open the hoards of the earth for his liberator. After that, he decided to fulfill any three wishes his liberator would express. When still nothing happened, he finally vowed to slay whoever would release him. Now this, Bettelheim says, reflects exactly the feelings of a young child temporarily left alone by his mother. At first, the child is simply hoping for his mother to return, thinking how sweet he will be towards her and how he will reward her. After a while, however, he becomes violently angry and starts fantasizing about the revenge he will take. The childish perception of time, too, is reflected in the story: to children, a mother's short absence seems "like ages." And just as the genie is locked in the jar, so the child's feelings, deprived of their object (mother), are "bottled up." These parallels allow the child to externalize, and to some extent clarify, the feelings of fear and anger that he experiences but that he neither fully understands nor wishes to accept. A child lacks sufficient distance from himself and his situation to face up to his emotions. He will not and cannot acknowledge his urge to destroy the person on whom he depends most; to do so would be too unsettling. "The Fisherman and the Jinny" provides the child with a less frightening outlet for his emotions.

There is more. The story allows the child to fantasize about outsmarting an adult, just as the fisherman got the better of the much more powerful Jinny. Admittedly, this fantasy is not only reassuring but also potentially disturbing. If adults can be outsmarted, then the child's parents might not be reliable protectors. The fairy tale's fantastic nature, however, makes it possible to circumvent this threat. As genies do not exist, the child can derive comfort from their defeat without losing confidence in real people. In addition, the child may cast, not himself, but a parent in the role of the fisherman. This, too, allows him to keep faith in his father and mother as protectors.

The story contains yet two other hidden messages. Only the fourth time around does the fisherman catch anything of significance. By including his three unsuccessful attempts (which, as far as the plot is concerned, might just as well have been left out) the story indirectly demonstrates the importance of perseverance. Furthermore, the fisherman's four efforts are set in contrast to the four stages of the Jinny's emotional development. Whereas the Jinny simply gives in to what he happens to be feeling, the fisherman remains calm and manages to overcome his disappointments. In this way, the story subtly "addresses the crucial problem which life early presents to all of us: whether to be governed by our emotions or by our rationality."[36]

As we have seen, fairy tales may contain not just one but *several* unconscious messages. This is important in Bettelheim's view because it allows children to respond to what preoccupies them and to ignore what they are not yet ready for. Not striking a chord, such premature meanings will simply go unnoticed. Perhaps even more than other forms of fiction, fairy tales speak in different ways to readers or listeners of different age groups.

Often, the unconscious messages contained in one and the same fairy tale are contradictory. In the case of "The Fisherman and the Jinny," for instance, children can empathize with the imprisoned Jinny and bemoan his fate, but they can also identify with the fisherman and rejoice in his victory. What is more, they can gain psychological comfort from both during one and the same reading. As embodiments of unconscious meanings, Bettelheim stresses, fairy tales are bound to be full of contradictions, as these also coexist in the unconscious mind itself.

Many parents feel uncomfortable about the unreal and irrational nature of fairy tales. They are concerned that young children might not be able to distinguish clearly between fiction and reality, or that they might become overfed by fantasies. This concern, according to Bettelheim, is unfounded. Both unprejudiced observation and scientific research show that children do *not* remain caught up in their fantasies. Moreover, to insist that children should be given only "truthful" pictures of the world is to ignore both their emotional needs and the fact that their minds work differently from those of adults. The only children who do withdraw from the world are children with an *underdeveloped* fantasy life: "those who live completely in their fantasies are beset by compulsive ruminations which rotate eternally around some narrow, stereotypical topics."[37] Children need a plurality of fantasies to put their emotions into a manageable shape, and to try out solutions to their inner conflicts.

Bettelheim also addresses the concerns that people have about the scary and violent nature of fairy tales. Children, it is often argued, should not be confronted with all too frightening subjects such as death, destruction, and aggression. What is more, reading or listening to such nasty stories can put dangerous ideas into their heads. Much better to let children grow up in their innocent childish world. And if there are to be stories with monsters, then these monsters should at least be benevolent and exhibit positive qualities. However, as psychoanalysis has taught us, childhood is not innocent. The plea for so-called safe stories ignores "the monster a child knows best and is most concerned with: the monster he feels or fears himself to be."[38] Parents who wish to protect their children from "monstrous" fantasies deny them an important way of mastering their primitive urges, *which are there no matter what.*

The relevance of this insight extends beyond the study of fairy tales; the parallels between the criticism of scary and violent fairy tales and that of certain television series and movies are obvious. Bettelheim's discussion of this issue therefore deserves to be quoted in full:

> In child or adult, the unconscious is a powerful determinant of behavior. When the unconscious is repressed and its content denied entrance into awareness, then eventually the person's conscious mind will be partially overwhelmed by derivatives of these unconscious elements, or else he is forced to keep such rigid, compulsive control over them that his personality may become severely crippled. But when unconscious material *is* to some degree permitted to come to awareness and worked through in imagination, its potential for causing harm — to ourselves or others — is much reduced; some of its forces can then be made to serve positive purposes. However, the prevalent parental belief is that a child must be diverted from what troubles him most: his formless, nameless anxieties, and his chaotic, angry, and even violent fantasies. Many parents believe that only conscious reality or pleasant and wish-fulfilling images should be presented to the child — that he should be exposed only to the sunny side of things. But such one-sided fare nourishes the mind only in a one-sided way, and real life is not all sunny.

There is a widespread refusal to let children know that the source of much that goes wrong in life is due to our very own natures — the propensity of all men for acting aggressively, asocially, selfishly, out of anger and anxiety. Instead, we want our children to believe that, inherently, all men are good. But children know that *they* are not always good; and often, even when they are, they would prefer not to be. This contradicts what they are told by their parents, and therefore makes the child a monster in his own eyes.

The dominant culture wishes to pretend, particularly where children are concerned, that the dark side of man does not exist, and professes a belief in an optimistic meliorism [this is what in chapter 3 I called *evolutionary utopianism*]. Psychoanalysis itself is viewed as having the purpose of making life easy — but this is not what its founder intended. Psychoanalysis was created to enable man to accept the problematic nature of life without being defeated by it, or giving in to escapism. Freud's prescription is that only by struggling against what seem like overwhelming odds can man succeed in wringing meaning out of his existence.[39]

Fairy tales, then, are important because they help the child to give vent to mental tension. Of course there are other ways of achieving this. All children play with toys, and in doing so literally *play out* their unconscious preoccupations. Many older girls are fascinated by horses, a hobby to which they often devote most of their spare time. This too, according to Bettelheim, constitutes the enactment of an unconscious preoccupation — in this case, of the girl's emotional need to control her own (sexually) animalistic drives. In addition, like reading or listening to fairy tales, such activities stimulate the child's imagination. That is to say, children can spin subjective fantasies around toys and horses in the same way that they bring their own subjective associations to, and subjectively elaborate on, fairy tales. This allows each child to work unconscious pressure out of his system in his own way.

Notwithstanding these similarities, Bettelheim says, fairy tales are special in one important respect. Playing with toys, children are able to act out their inner conflicts, but not to imagine possible ways out. They can only invent stories based on where they are, not stories that show them where they need to go. Fairy-tale stories, by contrast, also offer possible *resolutions* to inner conflicts. They teach the child, educate him;

and because they often do so in an indirect, nonmoralistic fashion, they are particularly effective.

Fairy tales have one other advantage — their universality. They are not the "personal expression of the unconscious and the experience of a particular person," but the "imaginary form that more or less universal human problems have attained as a story has been passed on over generations."[40] Although permitting subjective associations and elaborations, they deal with conflicts that are those of all humanity. They therefore speak to any and every child. To illustrate this universal nature, and to exemplify once more the interpretive insights psychoanalysis can provide, I wish to have a closer look at Bettelheim's analysis of "Snow White."

The most fundamental challenge that all human beings are faced with in their childhood is the question of how to manage the relationship with their parents, and the Oedipal problems connected to it. According to Bettelheim, this question therefore also plays a major role in many fairy tales. Among his examples is "Schneewittchen," the Brothers Grimm's version of the story of Snow White.

The first paragraph of "Schneewittchen," Bettelheim says, immediately sets out the story's main motif, the clash of sexual innocence and sexual desire.

> Once upon a time, in the middle of winter when the snow flakes fell like feathers from the sky, a queen sat at a window which had a frame of black ebony. And as she was sewing while looking at the snow, she pricked her finger with the needle and three drops of blood fell on the snow. The red looked so beautiful on the white snow that she thought to herself, "I wish I had a child as white as snow, as red as the blood, and with hair as black as the wood of the window frame." Soon after she got a little daughter who was as white as snow, as red as blood, and had hair as black as ebony, and she was therefore called Snow White. And when the child had been born, the queen died. After a year had passed, the king took himself another wife.[41]

The color white traditionally symbolizes chastity; red blood stands for carnality (the bleeding of menstruation, of the breaking of the hymen, and of childbirth). The clash of these two is acted out both between Snow White and her stepmother, and within Snow White herself.

The conflict between daughter and stepmother erupts first. As Snow White matures, the Queen becomes jealous of her and decides to have her killed. There are three aspects to this that in Bettelheim's view are significant from a psychoanalytic point of view. First, it is the stepmother, not the mother, who is jealous. The mother is written out of the story right away. And although the story makes it clear that the jealousy is rooted in a competition centered on physical attraction, there is no mention of any male for whose attention the two might be vying. Viewed psychoanalytically, the replacement of the mother and the absence of a desired male point to a censorship process similar to the one found in dreams; a process aimed at obscuring the Oedipal constellation that sets the story in motion. That the relationship of stepmother and daughter is indeed Oedipal in nature is apparent from the Queen's desperate desire to be more attractive than Snow White, and from her decision to get rid of her competitor. This is the second aspect to which Bettelheim draws attention: the Queen's jealousy, starting as it does only when Snow White begins to mature, is sexually motivated.

There is yet another, more hidden indication of the story's Oedipal character — the third aspect that Bettelheim highlights. From a psychoanalytic point of view, the Queen's decision to have Snow White killed is not only an expression of her own Oedipally determined desires. It can also be interpreted as symbolizing *Snow White's* Oedipal feelings. That is to say, the objective danger Snow White is in can be interpreted as a narrative representation of her (and indeed every child's) subjective wishes and fears. This may seem illogical. After all, the story states that Snow White really *is* in danger. As we have seen, however, such apparent contradictions are typical of fairy tales. The fairy-tale structure is not based on logical reasoning, but on the psychological workings of the unconscious. Looked at from this perspective, the Queen's murderous wishes reveal themselves as being a kind of narrative projection, a displacement of Snow White's own jealous and aggressive feelings (towards her stepmother) onto her stepmother. Moreover, a child who is dimly aware of such feelings may well feel that her parents have a right to banish her. This provides yet another psychological explanation for this aspect of the story.

As Bettelheim points out, the motif of the magic mirror blurs the distinction between the Queen and Snow White still further. When the Queen poses the question *Spieglein, Spieglein an der Wand, wer ist die Schönste im ganzen Land?* (Mirror, mirror on the wall, who is the fairest of them all?), at first the answer is: it is you. This reflects the picture a little girl has of her mother. When Snow White is older, the mirror tells the Queen that her daughter is *tausendmal schöner* than she is. Here, too, the Queen appears to see herself through Snow White's eyes. "A mother may be dismayed when looking into the mirror; she compares herself to her daughter and thinks to herself: 'My daughter is more beautiful than I am.' But the mirror says: 'She is a thousand times more beautiful' — a statement much more akin to an adolescent's exaggeration which he makes to enlarge his advantages and silence his inner voice of doubt."[42]

Although Snow White is not free from unconscious desires, initially her sexuality remains dormant (as with all children). Using the word *sexual* in its conventional, non-Freudian sense, one can therefore say that "Schneewittchen" is first evolved through a conflict between a sexually mature stepmother and a sexually innocent daughter. As the story unfolds, however, the focus shifts to the daughter; that is, to the conflict between sexual desire and sexual innocence within Snow White herself.

After having been left alone in the woods by the hunter who had been ordered to kill her, Snow White runs around aimlessly until she comes upon a little house. Hungry and tired, she enters, eats something from each of the seven plates standing on the table, and falls asleep in one of the seven beds, to be found by the seven dwarves, the occupants of the house. The kind-hearted dwarves allow Snow White to stay on condition that she keeps house for them. Snow White accepts, and from then on she cooks, makes the beds, washes, and performs all other household duties. This stay with the dwarves, Bettelheim asserts, represents a period of apprenticeship: Snow White learns the value of hard work, of discipline, and of sharing with others. But, he says, it is also the period her sexuality awakens. This becomes apparent when Snow White, instead of lying down on the floor, decides to sleep in one of the seven beds. As she knows full well that someone else will also want to sleep there, it is hard to escape the conclusion that unconsciously she wants to be in bed with someone else.

After this telling event, Snow White's inner conflict between childish innocence and sexual desire deepens. This is made clear by Snow White's inability to resist her stepmother's temptations. Three times the Queen puts on a disguise and visits her daughter, offering her first stay-laces, then a comb, and finally an apple — all erotic symbols. Each time, Snow White is taken in and falls victim to the objects' magic powers. Now the first two times, she is saved by the dwarves. Once having eaten from the poisoned apple, however, she is beyond their help. Why should this be so? The stay-laces and the comb represent Snow White's wish to be sexually attractive. The apple, of which Snow White moreover eats the *red* part, symbolizes something which goes beyond that. It stands for adult sexual lust. (One only needs to think of the apple with which Eve seduced Adam.) This demonstrates that Snow White is no longer a little girl, and has physically matured. She has outgrown the way of life she shared with the seven dwarves.

As Bettelheim puts it, the dwarves "are satisfied with an identical round of activities," and this "lack of change or of any desire for it is what makes their existence parallel that of the prepubertal child."[43] This is the life to which Snow White reverts after her first two forays into maturity. But human development cannot be postponed indefinitely, and Snow White is forced to leave this static, incomplete form of existence behind.

Although Snow White is now physically an adult, she "is by no means intellectually and emotionally ready for adulthood, as represented by marriage. Considerable growth and time are needed before the new, more mature personality is formed."[44] This is symbolized by Snow White's deathlike sleep in the glass coffin. What seems like mere passivity is actually a period of inner growth, just as in real life both children and adults need time on their own for reflection and meditation. The contemplative nature of this phase in Snow White's life is underlined by the three birds that visit her: the owl (wisdom), the raven (mature consciousness), and the dove (love). After this period of gestation Snow White is ready for a mature relationship — ready for her prince.

Whereas Snow White achieves inner harmony, her stepmother fails to do so. Unable to integrate the social and the antisocial aspects of human nature, she remains enslaved to her desires and gets caught up in an Oedipal competition with her daughter from which she cannot extricate herself. This imbalance between her contradictory drives proves to be her undoing: at the end of the story, at Snow White's wedding, she is forced to step into red-hot iron shoes, and has to dance until she drops dead on the floor. Through negative as well as positive exemplification, then, "Snow White" tells us that "adulthood can be reached only when these inner contradictions are resolved and a new awakening of the mature ego is achieved, in which red and white coexist harmoniously."[45]

Notes

[1] William Shakespeare, *Hamlet,* ed. Harold Jenkins, The Arden Shakespeare (London: Methuen, 1982). All references are to act, scene, and lines.

[2] Ernest Jones, *Hamlet and Oedipus* (New York/London: W. W. Norton, 1976).

[3] Jones, *Hamlet and Oedipus,* 54. By way of comparison, Jones quotes from Wilhelm Wetz's observations on *Othello:* "Nothing proves so well how false are the motives with which Iago tries to persuade himself as *the constant change in these motives*" (54–55).

[4] Jones, *Hamlet and Oedipus,* 55.

[5] Jones, *Hamlet and Oedipus,* 51–52.

[6] Claudius's crime cannot, of course, be the reason either. At the time of the outburst referred to, Hamlet has not yet been told by the ghost that Claudius is a murderer.

[7] Freud presupposes traditional family relations and role patterns here and moreover looks at things from a one-sidedly "male" perspective in that he sees the child's development primarily through a boy's (rather than a girl's) eyes. This bias has been justifiably criticized, notably by feminist scholars. Here, however, is not the place to enter upon a discussion of this issue; the present study is directed only towards elucidating in general terms the type of literary criticism that psychoanalysis implies.

[8] David Stafford-Clark, *What Freud Really Said* (Harmondsworth: Penguin, 1992), 105.

[9] In this process, Freud ascribes a major role to what he terms *Kastrationsangst,* castration anxiety. Seeing his little sister naked, the boy interprets her lack of a penis as the result of a punishment meted out by their father and, fearing that the same fate might befall him, represses his Oedipal feelings. This is a dubious concept in itself, and a good example of Freud's male bias.

[10] Jones, *Hamlet and Oedipus,* 76.

[11] This is a common pun, the first part of *country* suggesting a more vulgar word.

[12] Jones, *Hamlet and Oedipus,* 88.

[13] Jones, *Hamlet and Oedipus,* 91.

[14] Jones, *Hamlet and Oedipus,* 86.

[15] Jones, *Hamlet and Oedipus,* 50.

[16] Jones, *Hamlet and Oedipus,* 101.

[17] All this makes it even more surprising that Freud — contrary to Jones and rather to Jones's embarrassment — later in life came to support the view that the plays and poems attributed to Shakespeare were in reality written by Edward de Vere, seventeenth earl of Oxford.

[18] Sigmund Freud, *The Interpretation of Dreams*, trans. James Strachey, ed. James Strachey and Angela Richards, vol. 4 of *The Penguin Freud Library*, ed. Angela Richards and Albert Dickson (Harmondsworth: Penguin, 1991), 368.

[19] Jones, *Hamlet and Oedipus*, 51.

[20] Jones, *Hamlet and Oedipus*, 129–30.

[21] Jones, *Hamlet and Oedipus*, 141.

[22] Heinrich Heine, *Historisch-kritische Gesamtausgabe der Werke*, ed. Manfred Windfuhr (Hamburg: Hoffmann und Campe, 1973), 206, 208; and Leonard Forster, ed., *The Penguin Book of German Verse*, rev. ed. (Harmondsworth: Penguin, 1959), 328–29.

[23] Walter Schönau, "Literarisches Lesen in psychoanalytischer Sicht," in *Freiburger literaturpsychologische Gespräche* 4 (1985): 9–26, and *Einführung in die psychoanalytische Literaturwissenschaft*, Sammlung Metzler 259 (Stuttgart: Metzler, 1991), 43–45.

[24] To avoid misunderstanding, Schönau is not saying that it is possible to interpret the various people and events in Heine's poetry simply on the basis of his biography, as the early studies on Heine sought to do. Heine's poetry is not an artistic duplication of reality, but fiction. Schönau's point is that irrespective of its *biographical* realism, or lack thereof, Heine's fiction has specific *psychological* roots. (In this respect, literary fantasies are similar to nonliterary, everyday fantasies.)

[25] Gerhard Höhn, *Heine-Handbuch. Zeit, Person, Werk*, 2nd rev. ed. (Stuttgart/Weimar: Metzler, 1997), 64.

[26] Sigmund Freud, *The Origins of Religion*, trans. James Strachey, ed. Albert Dickson, vol. 13 of *The Penguin Freud Library*, ed. Angela Richards and Albert Dickson (Harmondsworth: Penguin, 1990), 221; quoted in Schönau, *Einführung in die psychoanalytische Literaturwissenschaft*, 43–44.

[27] Schönau, "Literarisches Lesen in psychoanalytischer Sicht," 20.

[28] The following account is based on Höhn, *Heine-Handbuch*, 60–64.

[29] Here, an additional explanation for Heine's framing of the Lore-Ley story is to be found. The introduction of the subjective framework marks the modern poet's inability to adopt Romantic motifs in an unreflecting manner. (The Lore-Ley story is not really an old-time fairy tale but a Romantic invention.)

[30] Höhn, *Heine-Handbuch*, 60.

[31] Höhn, *Heine-Handbuch*, 64.

[32] Bruno Bettelheim, *The Uses of Enchantment: The Meaning and Importance of Fairy Tales* (Harmondsworth: Penguin, 1991).

[33] Bettelheim, *Uses of Enchantment*, 49.

[34] Bettelheim, *Uses of Enchantment*, 6.

[35] Bettelheim, *Uses of Enchantment*, 28–29.

[36] Bettelheim, *Uses of Enchantment*, 33.

[37] Bettelheim, *Uses of Enchantment*, 119.

[38] Bettelheim, *Uses of Enchantment*, 120.

[39] Bettelheim, *Uses of Enchantment*, 7–8.

[40] Bettelheim, *Uses of Enchantment*, 58.

[41] Bettelheim, *Uses of Enchantment*, 202.

[42] Bettelheim, *Uses of Enchantment*, 207.

[43] Bettelheim, *Uses of Enchantment*, 210.

[44] Bettelheim, *Uses of Enchantment*, 213.

[45] Bettelheim, *Uses of Enchantment*, 214.

5: The Psychoanalysis of Culture

IN THE PREVIOUS CHAPTER, the focus was on the interpretation of individual works of fiction. In the present chapter, I wish to examine the application of psychoanalysis to a number of social phenomena. My point of departure will be Freud's *Totem und Tabu* (Totem and Taboo, 1913).

Totem and Taboo I

Totem und Tabu ranks as one of Freud's least convincing works. One of its early critics, the American anthropologist A. L. Kroeber, who was by no means unsympathetic towards psychoanalysis, considered it to be so weak that he compared demolishing it to breaking a butterfly on the wheel.[1] Academic opinion of the book has hardly improved since. Yet *Totem und Tabu* has had a strong influence on literary circles, in particular on German writers of the first half of the twentieth century. Moreover, although the theory it develops may be untenable, the book has proved a source of thought-provoking social critique. Before assessing its merits and demerits, however, let us look at its main ideas.

Totem und Tabu aims to apply the findings of psychoanalysis to certain unsolved problems of anthropology. Central to this aim are two key elements of prehistoric and, in Freud's terminology, "primitive" societies, totems and taboos. Totemism, Freud explains on the basis of the anthropological theories of his day (especially those of J. G. Frazer and W. Robertson Smith) and with reference to the native tribes of Australia, his main object of research, is a kind of prereligious system of belief and the basis of prehistoric and "primitive" social organization.

> Australian tribes fall into smaller divisions, or clans, each of which is named after its totem. What is a totem? It is as a rule an animal (whether edible and harmless or dangerous and feared), which stands in a peculiar relation to the whole clan. In the first place, the totem is the common ancestor [*Stammvater*] of the clan; at the same time it is

their guardian spirit and helper, which sends them oracles and, if dangerous to others, recognizes and spares its own children. Conversely, the clansmen are under a sacred obligation (subject to automatic sanctions) not to kill or destroy their totem and to avoid eating its flesh (or deriving benefit from it in other ways).[2]

It is only at special occasions — holy festivals — that this obligation is temporarily lifted. Through such special totem meals the bond that unites the clan members with each other and with their totem is reconfirmed and strengthened.

The totem is subject to specific taboos. A taboo "is principally expressed in prohibitions and restrictions. Our collocation 'holy dread' would often coincide in meaning with 'taboo.'"[3] The restrictions connected with a taboo

> are distinct from religious or moral prohibitions. They are not based upon any divine ordinance, but may be said to impose themselves. They differ from moral prohibitions in that they do not fall into a system that declares that certain abstinences are necessary and gives reasons for that necessity. Taboo prohibitions have no grounds and are of unknown origin. Though they are unintelligible to *us*, by those who are dominated by them they are taken as a matter of course.[4]

The two most important totemistic taboos are, first, the prohibition against the killing of the totem animal and, second, the prohibition against sexual intercourse with members of the same clan. This second taboo is the "notorious and mysterious"[5] exogamy (literally, marriage outside one's own clan), which Freud takes as resulting from a powerful fear of incest.

As I said, Freud's declared aim is to shed some light on these peculiar archaic phenomena by confronting them with the insights of psychoanalysis. What this confrontation shows him is that the way prehistoric and "primitive" peoples behave towards their totems is essentially similar to the obsessive behavior of his neurotic patients. Hence the subtitle of his book, *Einige Übereinstimmungen im Seelenleben der Wilden und der Neurotiker* (Some Points of Agreement between the Mental Lives of Savages and Neurotics). But what exactly does this similarity consist in? Like prehistoric and "primitive" peoples, neurotics obey a number of commands and prohibitions that to an outsider appear completely unnecessary and groundless. They can only walk on specific parts of the pavement, for example, or are unable to touch anything red. As with taboos, these obsessional commands and prohibitions tend to get extended from one object or person to another that in the eyes of the neurotic is related to it; neurotics behave as if the forbidden objects or persons were "carriers of a dangerous infection liable to be spread by contact on to everything in their neighbourhood."[6] By way of illustration, Freud compares the behavior of a Maori chief (an example he borrows from J. G. Frazer) to that of one of his neurotic patients:

> "A Maori chief would not blow a fire with his mouth; for his sacred breath would communicate its sanctity to the fire, which would pass it on to the pot, which would pass it on to the man who ate the meat, which was in the pot, which stood on the fire, which was breathed on by the chief; so that the eater, infected by the chief's breath conveyed through these intermediaries, would surely die."
>
> My patient's husband purchased a household article of some kind and brought it home with him. She insisted that it should be removed or it would make the rooms she lived in "impossible." For she had heard that the article had been bought in a shop situated in, let us say, "Smith" Street. "Smith," however, was the married name of a woman friend of hers who lived in a distant town and whom she had known in her youth under her maiden name. This friend of hers was at the moment "impossible" or taboo. Consequently the article that had been purchased here in Vienna was as taboo as the friend herself with whom she must not come into contact.[7]

Finally, again as with taboos, obsessional prohibitions can be lifted, or their transgression atoned for, by certain "ritual" actions such as washing one's hands or walking on the right part of the pavement twice.

The key characteristic of obsessive behavior, Freud says, is its *ambivalent* nature. Neurotics erect barriers to actions that they consciously abhor but unconsciously desire. The barriers are so high, and they obsess the neurotic so much, precisely because his unconscious wish to perform the tabooed action is so powerful. This thesis may seem odd at first. Why should anyone have, say, an unconscious desire to walk on specific parts of the pavement, consciously abhor doing this, and then impose a taboo on this action? The mystery disappears when we take into account that most obsessional prohibitions are the result of displacement, or even of a series of displacements. Frustrated wishes get displaced, attach themselves to objects (*Ersatzobjekte,* surrogate objects) which are, in the unconscious mind of the neurotic, related to the original wished-for object; and the barrier (the taboo) usually follows the displaced wish like a shadow. The manifest constellation of object and wish is thus as a rule different from the latent, original one.

Now if the way prehistoric and "primitive" peoples behave towards their totems and the way neurotics behave are essentially similar, and if neurotic behavior is grounded in ambivalence, then — Freud suggests — totemistic behavior must be ambivalent too. He uses this insight in two ways.

First, Freud tackles a number of specific problems with which the anthropology of his day was grappling. Let us look at one of them. For prehistoric and "primitive" peoples, the dead are taboo. Touching the dead or even being close to them is dangerous; the bereaved are placed under quarantine for a certain period of time; pronouncing the names of the dead is often forbidden; and so on. The reason seems to be that those who die are thought to become demons, intent on harming the living.[8] But why should this happen? Why should the deceased suddenly turn into demons? His insight into the ambivalent roots of neurotic symptoms allows Freud to answer this question. When someone loses a partner or a beloved friend, he is often plagued by feelings of guilt. Objectively innocent of the other's death, he yet blames himself for it. The psychoanalytic study of these puzzling self-accusations, which to an outsider are completely unnecessary and groundless, has shown the reason for this. Such obsessive self-reproaches result from the fact that, with a smaller or larger part of his unconscious mind, the survivor actually willed the beloved's death. For however much we may love someone, there is always an unconscious countertendency; no strong feelings are ever free from ambivalence. The survivor's self-reproaches are based, not on what he consciously did, but on what he unconsciously desired. The same process, according to Freud, can be observed with prehistoric and "primitive" peoples, with one important difference: the hostile feelings against the deceased, instead of becoming the source of obsessive self-reproaches, are projected onto the deceased. "The hostility, of which the survivors know nothing and moreover wish to know nothing, is ejected from internal perception into the external world, and thus detached from them and pushed on to someone else."[9] Through this unconscious process, the erstwhile beloved are transformed into malicious demons.

Freud's second project is more ambitious. In the final and, as it turned out, most influential part of *Totem und Tabu,* he develops a historical theory to explain the origins of the two most important totemistic taboos, the prohibition against the killing of the totem and the prohibition against sexual intercourse between members of the same clan (that is, against incest). What is more, the theory is also meant to explain the origins of the Oedipus complex and even of society as a whole. Freud's starting-point is Darwin's hypothesis of the primal horde: the hypothesis that in its earliest state society was a mere horde, led by a tyrannical, violent, and jealous father who kept all the women to himself and oppressed the sons. On the basis of this hypothesis and with the so-called totem meal at the back of his mind, Freud erects a highly speculative historical theory. One day, he conjectures, the brothers got together, killed the father and, being cannibals, ate him. After they had killed him, however, remorse set in, for the brothers' feelings towards their father were — like all powerful human feelings — ambivalent. The brothers hated and envied the father, but they also loved and admired him.

> The dead father became stronger than the living one had been — for events took the same course we so often see them follow in human affairs to this day. What up to then had been prevented by his actual existence was thenceforward prohibited by the sons themselves, in accordance with the psychological procedure so familiar to us in psychoanalyses under the name of "deferred obedience."[10] They revoked their deed by forbidding the killing of the totem, the substitute for their father; and they renounced its fruits by resigning their claim to the women who had now been set free. They thus created out of their filial sense of guilt the two fundamental taboos of totemism, which for that very reason inevitably correspond to the two wishes of the Oedipus complex.[11]

The totem, then, acted as a surrogate for the father. By venerating it, the brothers atoned for their feelings of guilt. "The totemistic system was, as it were, a covenant with their father, in which he promised them everything that a childish imagination may expect from a father — protection, care and indulgence — while on their side they undertook to respect his life, that is to say, not to repeat the deed which had brought destruction on their real father."[12] The renunciation of the women, too, was an expression of guilt and furthermore prevented the kind of sexually motivated infighting that had led to the killing of the father. In order to preserve the highly unstable social equilibrium that had been achieved, the two original totemistic taboos were gradually amplified into a whole system of moral restrictions. Over time, totemistic veneration developed into a "real" religion, the surrogate father having acquired an ever-stronger, divine status. Finally, the killing of the primal father was *artistically* assimilated, the most important traces of which are to be found in the various Oedipal (Hamletean) stories in mythology and literature. Therefore, Freud boldly concludes, it is in the killing of the primal father that "the beginnings of religion, morals, society and art"[13] can be found.

Totem and Taboo II:
Its Problems and Its Influence on Literature

As I mentioned earlier, *Totem und Tabu* has found little favor with anthropologists. It is not hard to understand why. Even at the basic level of logic and argument the book is seriously flawed. For example, if the brothers in the primal horde renounced the women, how did they procreate? Does Freud's theory not imply that there were other hordes as well? If so, did they too experience a primal killing? If not, how can *their* beliefs and precepts be explained? There is no point in completing the list of argumentative gaps; they are plain for everyone to see. Instead, I want to draw attention to a number of presuppositions that underlie Freud's historico-anthropological speculations and whose problematic nature is perhaps less apparent. To begin with, several assumptions that Freud takes over from anthropological studies of his time have today lost all plausibility. This applies even to key assumptions such as the idea that there exists a necessary relationship between totemism and exogamy, or the hypothesis of the primal horde. But there is more.

The central theory of *Totem und Tabu* — the theory of the primal killing and its consequences — is problematic not only from the viewpoint of contemporary anthropology but also from that of contemporary biology. As Freud himself acknowledges, this theory presupposes "the assumption of a collective mind, which makes it possible to neglect the interruptions of mental acts caused by the extinction of the individual."[14]

This collective mind, which according to Freud results partly from tradition and education and partly from "the inheritance of mental dispositions,"[15] is responsible for the fact that the guilty feelings generated by the primal killing remained active even in generations for whom this deed no longer possessed tangible reality.

Now the assumption of the existence of such a collective human psyche and especially the biological twist that Freud gives it are highly questionable. Here Freud seems to have fallen victim to the influence of Lamarckism. Based on ideas developed by the French biologist Jean Lamarck (1744–1829), which gained popularity during the late nineteenth and early twentieth centuries, this theory propounded that acquired traits can be inherited, that for example emotions and attitudes such as guilt, arrogance, and greed can become part of a person's biological make-up and be transmitted biologically to his children. Lamarckism, however, has been disproved by modern genetics. But even if we accepted the possibility of a collective human psyche as a socially, rather than biologically, produced phenomenon, how is this social production supposed to take place? After all, the collective psyche Freud is thinking of is unconscious, whereas tradition and education are commonly thought of as the transfer of *conscious* meanings. Not that it is far-fetched to assume that tradition and education also transfer unconscious contents. But to erect a whole theory on this assumption seems to me only admissible if it explains exactly how this happens. Freud provides no such explanation.

Finally, the central theory of *Totem und Tabu* is problematic even from the perspective of psychoanalysis itself. As we saw both in part 1 and in chapter 4, psychoanalysis typically looks at mental and social phenomena from the perspective of their psychological relevance. Psychoanalysis is a *functionalistic* theory; it explains mental and social phenomena by reference to the psychological function they fulfill for the people who produce them (as authors do in the case of literary texts), use them (as readers of literary texts do), or benefit from them in some other way. This is different from *Totem und Tabu,* or at least from the central theory it expounds. Here, the presupposition seems to be that to explain a phenomenon is to uncover, not its psychological function, but its historical roots.

The difference between the methodological thrust of psychoanalysis and the historical theory offered by *Totem und Tabu* is not absolute, for the historical roots that Freud uncovers are discussed in functionalistic terms (atonement for murder, need for social stability, and so on). Still, the difference is striking enough to require an explanation. Why, then, did Freud move away from his usual approach?

The first reason that suggests itself is that he fell victim to the scientific ideals of his academic education. His university teachers — internationally renowned physiologists, biologists, and psychiatrists such as Ernst Wilhelm von Brücke and Theodor Meynert — adhered to *positivism*, the view that science consists in the methodical interrelating of objectively given, material, measurable phenomena. Freud held on to this view even during his postdoctoral research. Only when he began to develop psychoanalysis did he abandon the one-sided emphasis on the material nature of the phenomena he was trying to explain in favor of a more inclusive view of science, a view that recognized the autonomy and thus the scientific relevance of "immaterial," only indirectly observable, *mental* phenomena. But Freud never completely overcame his old positivistic leanings, which from time to time reasserted themselves. It seems likely that this happened in the case of *Totem und Tabu* as well. Working on extinct and "primitive" societies he had never seen and thus having to operate with highly uncertain data and speculative anthropological theories, Freud's old positivistic conscience started nagging, and induced him to look for hard, observable facts. The irony is, of course, that the hard, observable facts with which Freud explains the origins of religion, morality, society, and art are much more speculative than a purely psychological explanation would have been.

The second reason why Freud was so enamored with the idea of the killing of the primal father can be found by applying the insights of psychoanalysis to *Totem und Tabu;* that is, by looking at the relationship between this text and Freud in the same way that psychoanalytic literary criticism looks at the relationship between text and author.[16] When working on the four texts published together in 1913 as *Totem und Tabu,* Freud was faced with two major developments. For one thing, the psychoanalytic movement was entering its first phase of institutionalization. The International Psycho-Analytical Association and a number of psychoanalytic journals were founded, conferences were being organized, factions started to emerge. For another, several admirers and supporters of psychoanalysis now turned their backs on it; the secession of Alfred Adler and Carl Gustav Jung, both of whom were to found schools of their own, hit Freud especially hard. It is not difficult to see the parallels between this situation and that described in *Totem und Tabu:* Freud, the father of psychoanalysis, in control of his movement; his sons (followers) who both admire and envy him; the killing (attack) of him by Jung and other followers; and finally the emergence of new beliefs (psychological theories) and institutions. From this perspective, it would appear that the central theory of *Totem und Tabu* was stimulated by an unconscious process of "Verschiebung,"[17] a displacement of Freud's own biographically specific preoccupations onto the object of his research.

Its serious shortcomings as an academic piece of work notwithstanding, *Totem und Tabu* had a strong influence on literature, especially on German literature of the 1920s and 1930s. Its influence is most clearly to be seen in the works of Thomas Mann (1875–1955).

Thomas Mann hit upon Freud's work in 1911.[18] In that year, he read Freud's interpretation of *Gradiva,* a novella by the Danish author Wilhelm Jensen. Jensen's novella and Freud's interpretation provided the inspiration for a novella of his own, *Der Tod in Venedig* (Death in Venice, 1912), the story of a writer whose repressed homosexual desires are reawakened when he falls in love with a beautiful Polish boy. Later, Thomas Mann would read a good deal more of Freud. But the initial inspiration — the *return of the repressed* — which had helped to clarify so many of his own intuitive ideas, would remain a key motif of his literary oeuvre. As it did for Freud, for Mann the ineradicability of the repressed pointed to the need for a balance between conscious and unconscious drives, between id and superego, between repressing and acting out. This insight, together with similar ones taken from the philosophies of Schopenhauer and Nietzsche, gave rise to the dichotomies that structure all Mann's novels and stories: those between artist and bourgeois, nature and culture, sexuality and abstinence, and so on. With the help of these psychoanalytically (and philosophically) inspired dichotomies, Thomas Mann portrayed the conflicts of his protagonists and exposed the repressive and all too often pharisaical side of their social surroundings. But Freud provided Mann with more than a descriptive psychology and a means to penetrate the bourgeois surface of respectability. It is here that *Totem und Tabu* comes in.

By opening up "ungeheure Perspektiven seelischer Vergangenheit, Urwelttiefen moralischer, gesellschaftlicher, mythisch-religiöser Früh- und Vorgeschichte der Menschheit" (the vast horizons of humanity's spiritual past, the primeval depths of its moral, social, and mythico- religious early history and prehistory),[19] *Totem und Tabu*, Thomas Mann felt, put man in touch again with his roots; with a long-forgotten, and perhaps in many ways uncanny, yet still relevant past. It made man aware of the ancient foundations of civilization, the awesome forces behind his well-ordered daily life, the unfathomable depth of his bureaucratic- technological world. At first sight, this may seem a rather obscurantist reading of *Totem und Tabu*. But Thomas Mann neither aimed at nor fell prey to any form of irrationalism. His seemingly metaphysical approach to man and society was not directed against enlightened, critical thinking but was an attempt to strengthen and amplify it. In his view, the mythical imagination helped man to address the social and political issues of the time in a more confident and more comprehensive way by providing him with a sense of tradition, of a common ancestry and a shared purpose, and by supplementing his critical faculties with a more emotional, em- pathetic type of intelligence.

For Mann, then, the mythical imagination was a progressive force. His fascination with Freud's study of prehistoric man was "keine Inbrust zur Vergangenheit um der Vergangenheit willen" (no ardor for the past for the sake of the past)[20] but stemmed from an active engagement with contemporary reality. This reality was shaped, above all, by the rise of National Socialism: Thomas Mann's interest in *Totem und Tabu* origi- nated in the 1920s and continued well into the 1930s. (The novel that shows this interest most clearly is the four-part *Joseph und seine Brüder* — Joseph and His Brothers — published between 1934 and 1943.) The Nazis of course had their own mythical imagination, and the main thrust of Mann's appropriation of Freud's study was directed precisely against their reactionary irrationalism. Mann used Freud's prehistoric "mythol- ogy" as a means to reclaim the romantic legacy hijacked by the Nazis and to put it in the service of a humanistic enterprise. His writing was an attempt to explore and indeed employ the power of myth without sur- rendering the power of reason.

Besides Thomas Mann there were other German writers who were fascinated by *Totem und Tabu*. Like Mann, they saw in its daring historical speculations a source of regeneration for the present. Unlike Mann, however, most of them read into the book a critique of the "decadence" of Western civilization. What resonated with them was the picture Freud painted — or rather the picture they thought he painted — of the natural, uninhibited, raw nature of man, of the vitalist "power man" that below the surface of cultural refinement still lived in all of us.[21] This reading of *Totem und Tabu* reduced Freud's analysis of complex interrelationships (between aggression and repression, transgression and remorse, mental processes and social developments) to the depiction of an original barbaric freedom. What resulted was a naïve glorification of man's primal instincts with strong Darwinist undertones. To take only one example, this is how Ernst Jünger (1895–1998) described man's true nature, as he saw it:

> The endless ancestral chain drags behind him; he is entwined and bound by myriad ties and invisible threads to the roots of the primeval swamp, whose fermenting heat first bred the seed from which he came. The ferocity, the brutality, the harsh colors of the urges may have been smoothed and tempered through all the millennia in which society has restrained impatient lusts and desires. Increasing refinement may have polished and elevated him. Yet in the essence of his being, the old impulse still slumbers. Veiled by social customs and good manners . . ., the animal within lives on. When the pendulum of life swings back to the red line of the primitive, then the mask drops away and primeval man, the cave-dweller, bursts out in his ancient nakedness, with all the unbridled force of his liberated urges. . . . In this struggle, the weak must perish whilst the victors, their weapons grasped more securely in their fists, stride forth across the bodies of the slain victims, further and deeper into the battle, into life.[22]

With many writers, it is not possible to distinguish clearly between the influence of *Totem und Tabu* and that of other anthropological and philosophical works that deal with similar topics. But there can be no doubt that in the 1920s and 1930s Freud's study was a considerable literary force.

Totem and Taboo III:
Its Application to the Study of Culture

Having examined both the shortcomings of *Totem und Tabu* and its impact on literature, we must now ask a further question. When so many of the things it says are wrong, and when its main influence has been on the creative imagination, what then is the analytic relevance of *Totem und Tabu*? At the beginning of this chapter, I maintained that the book has proved a source of thought-provoking social critique. So what does this critical potential consist in? What insights does *Totem und Tabu* provide for the analysis of contemporary society? I wish to answer this question by looking at two modern interpretations of Freud's study, those of Mario Erdheim and Odo Marquard.

In his introduction to a recent German edition of *Totem und Tabu,* the psychoanalyst and cultural historian Mario Erdheim proposes a reading of Freud's text that shifts the focus from its "exotic" subject-matter to what he sees as its underlying intention, the attempt to develop a psychoanalysis of culture.[23] The significance of Freud's text, Erdheim argues, lies not in its rather dubious contribution to cultural anthropology but in the way it links mental and social phenomena. *Totem und Tabu* is Freud's first major study aimed at rendering visible how unconscious mental processes determine social norms and values.

In other words, for Erdheim, Freud's investigation of prehistoric and "primitive" totems and taboos is not about a way of life that we have long since left behind. It is a case study of the unconscious roots of social dos and don'ts. Every society has its taboos, and Freud demonstrates that such intersubjectively shared manifestations of culture are just as open to psychoanalysis as are its more subjective manifestations such as literary texts. From this perspective, *Totem und Tabu* is first and foremost a further step in the way psychoanalysis subverts the dichotomies of normal/abnormal and healthy/pathological. In previous books and papers, Freud showed that it is not only hysterics, neurotics, and perverts who are subject to repression, antisocial urges, and other expressions of the unconscious but that *all* human beings are determined by the interplay of conscious and unconscious mental processes. Thus he uncovered the role of the unconscious in human sexuality, in dreams, in slips of the tongue and other faulty actions, in literature and art. With *Totem und*

Tabu, Freud devotes a whole study to the unconscious patterning of *culture,* to social (rather than individual) repressions, taboos, and prohibitions. In Erdheim's reading, then, *Totem und Tabu* is not about the earliest beginnings of culture, but about the unconscious foundations of culture. In this way, Erdheim manages to translate Freud's historico-anthropological approach into a functionalistic one and thus to recover the analytic relevance of *Totem und Tabu.*

To find out what this means in concrete terms let us examine one of Erdheim's examples, the way Germans deal with the National Socialist past. In Germany, National Socialism and its discussion are subject to a significant number of taboos. Some of these have even become law. Whereas in most other countries someone who denies the Holocaust simply tends to be regarded as a pathetic fool, in Germany the *Auschwitzlüge* (Auschwitz lie) is a criminal offense. Giving the Nazi salute, too, constitutes a criminal offense; a legal ban, incidentally, that neo-Nazis manage to dodge by giving the Nazi salute with their left arm. Other taboos become apparent only in special circumstances. For example, when in 1988 the then President of the German Parliament, Philipp Jenninger, devoted a large part of a major public speech to a reconstruction of the thought processes of the ordinary Germans who had supported Hitler in the 1930s, he faced a public outcry. To make his point, he had employed a number of rhetorical questions ("Had the Jews not overstepped the mark?") but it was clear, or should have been so, that he did not hold such views himself. He had continuously added phrases along the lines of "This, at least, is what people thought at the time." All the same, Jenninger was forced to resign. In Germany, it would seem, references to and discussions of National Socialism that appear even remotely understanding are completely taboo.

Freud's analysis of neurotic patients had taught him that their obsessional prohibitions were grounded in unconscious desires. His patients abhorred the prohibited act *and desired it at the same time.* "The prohibition owes its strength and its obsessive character precisely to its unconscious opponent, the concealed and undiminished desire."[24] In *Totem und Tabu,* Freud applied this insight to a cultural phenomenon, social taboos. Erdheim now takes the same approach. The taboos surrounding National Socialism, he suggests, spring from an unconscious fear that fascism might take root again. The levels of emotion generated by certain

ways of dealing with the National Socialist past, in particular by identifi-
catory and quasi-identificatory ones, the panicky speed with which people distance themselves from the "impossible" views, the *cordon sanitaire*
that is immediately drawn around the offender — all this is analogous to
the actions of neurotics, who behave as if the forbidden objects or persons were "carriers of a dangerous infection liable to be spread by contact on to everyone in their neighbourhood."[25] Deep down, it seems,
people are not convinced that they have really left the National Socialist
past behind. Unconsciously they seem to harbor, if not a direct wish to
transgress, then at least the nagging suspicion that they might not be
immune to the lure of transgression.[26]

But what about the central theory of *Totem und Tabu*? Freud's reflections on the relationship between mental processes and social taboos
may be applicable to contemporary society, but can his theory of the
killing of the primal father be used in a similar way? What is *its* contemporary relevance? These questions bring us to Odo Marquard's interpretation of *Totem und Tabu*.[27]

The German philosopher Odo Marquard interprets Freud's text not
as an investigation into a unique historical event that (supposedly) took
place in some distant past, but as an examination of the mental roots and
repercussions of social disobedience; as an examination of the *psychological structure of revolutions,* or at least a certain type of revolution. Just as
for Erdheim, for Marquard the analytic relevance of *Totem und Tabu* lies
in the insights it provides into the link between unconscious mental
phenomena and large-scale social phenomena.

The revolution to which Marquard applies these Freudian insights
is the German student revolution of the late 1960s. His thesis is that the
Studentenrevolution represents a form of inverted totemism, which can
be explained by an inverted concept of deferred obedience, a concept of
deferred *dis*obedience. How is this to be understood?

Up to a point, Marquard says, the clash between the students and
the world of their parents can simply be explained as resulting from a
generational conflict. Each new generation has it own norms and values,
which invariably leads to frictions with the previous generation. Taken
by itself, however, this explanation is insufficient. It accounts neither for
the scale and vehemence of the protests nor for the extent to which
society as a whole became the object of attack. The question according

to Marquard is therefore: why did this particular generational conflict assume such extreme proportions? The answer, he says, can be found in the students' mental disposition, their massive guilt complex based on their parents' failure to rise up against Hitler.

The Hitler period was largely free from rebellion. The vast majority of Germans had either played along with the National Socialist regime or had actively supported it. After the Second World War, the necessity to rebuild their heavily damaged country directed the German people's attention to the needs of the present, helping them to forget about the horrors of the past. *Erst kommt das Fressen, dann kommt die Moral* (Eating comes first; moral questions come later), Marquard says, quoting from Brecht's *Threepenny Opera*. Not until Germany's reconstruction — the economic miracle — had been achieved, did the situation change.

> Only once conditions were made materially tolerable, through the postwar reconstruction, and then brought to a level of surplus, did dismay with the horrors of the past fully reach the conscience of Germany, and only then, as it were by time-delay, did it become morally really intolerable.[28]

This manifested itself not with the members of the older generation, who by and large had rationalized or repressed their lack of courage (or worse) under National Socialism, but rather with their children. It was the younger generation that felt remorse and, as a result, wanted to atone for the sins of the past. This led them to rebel against what they saw as the continuation of fascism into the present.

This situation, Marquard argues, is the exact mirror image of the one described by Freud in *Totem und Tabu*. The students developed a guilty conscience, not (like the sons in the primal horde) about a rebellion committed by them, but about a rebellion not committed by their parents. The result therefore is not deferred (or subsequent) obedience, but *deferred (or subsequent) disobedience*. The "revolt against the dictator (the father of the 'fatherless society'[29]) which largely failed to take place between 1933 and 1945 was vicariously made up for in the rebellion against what had taken the place of the dictatorship after 1945."[30] The outcome was a form of *inverted totemism*. Totemism leads to pronounced sexual abstinence; inverted totemism leads to pronounced hedonism, which is why the student revolution was at the same time a sexual revolution. Totemism implies establishing social taboos; inverted totemism implies breaking them. Totemism is an attempt to preserve the social order; inverted totemism is an attempt to undermine it. Finally, the "fact that an action was omitted also now (belatedly) forces every thought to proceed immediately to action."[31] Hence inverted totemism is characterized, not by realistic restraint, but by idealistic zeal, by an activism blind to political, economic, and other constraints.

The students' disobedience — their rebellion — could of course be psychologically successful only if its object was identical or similar to that of their parents' obedience. That is to say, the students could assuage their guilty feelings only by making up for their parents' failure; and they could make up for their parents' failure only by doing now what their parents had failed to do then: by opposing fascism. "Because fascism was the target against which a revolt did not materialize then, today the target of the compensatory revolt must also be fascism."[32] This explains the students' absurd equation of capitalism with fascism, and of the Federal Republic with Hitler's Germany. The consumer society with its market economy was seen as controlling people from within by creating false needs. Marriage and similar institutions, the rebels believed, oppressed people by preventing them from expressing their true desires. Harmless popular entertainment was the expression of a so-called culture industry, distracting people from real social issues. Schools were instruments of indoctrination. Even liberal democracy itself, with its elections and freedom of speech, was seen as just another form of totalitarianism, a cunning way to prevent people from looking for (true) freedom beyond the existing system by giving them some (quasi-)freedom within it. Through this equation of democratic present and fascist past, the students managed to provide their wish to rebel with the adequate object.

The psychological mechanism that Marquard identifies as underlying the student revolution is a sophisticated one. It is not only *the fact that* the students did what the previous generation had failed to do but also *the way in which* they did it that helped them to ease their conscience. By indicting "the system" and its alleged representatives, they managed to avoid thinking about their own responsibilities and the extent to which they were living up to them (or were failing to do so). By consistently and vehemently accusing others, they recovered their moral purity; for if others are to blame, one must be innocent oneself. Marquard describes this as the flight from having a conscience into being the conscience of others (*Flucht aus dem Gewissenhaben in das Gewissensein*), as the self-deception that says "that one no longer needs to *have* a conscience — when it is overburdened by reproaches of guilt — if one can *be* the conscience." He concludes: "Deferred obedience gives rise to the kind of conscience that one *has,* but deferred *dis*obedience gives rise to the kind of conscience that one *is:* the tribunal that one evades by becoming it."[33]

Before assessing the validity of Marquard's ideas, let me summarize them with a diagram.

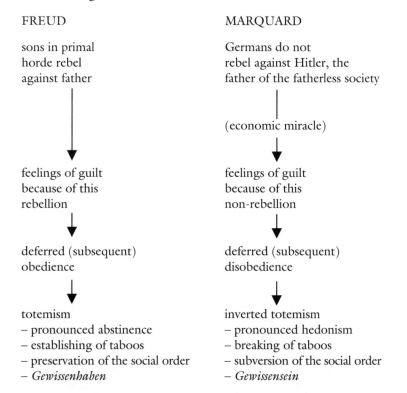

FREUD

sons in primal
horde rebel
against father

feelings of guilt
because of this
rebellion

deferred (subsequent)
obedience

totemism
– pronounced abstinence
– establishing of taboos
– preservation of the social order
– *Gewissenhaben*

MARQUARD

Germans do not
rebel against Hitler, the
father of the fatherless society

(economic miracle)

feelings of guilt
because of this
non-rebellion

deferred (subsequent)
disobedience

inverted totemism
– pronounced hedonism
– breaking of taboos
– subversion of the social order
– *Gewissensein*

How convincing are Marquard's ideas? At first sight, they may well seem to be flawed right from the start. After all, by explaining the German student revolution as the mirror image of the actions of the sons who killed the primal father, Marquard seems to be taking for granted precisely the most questionable historico-anthropological ideas of *Totem und Tabu*. On closer inspection, however, it becomes clear that this is not the case. What Marquard takes over from *Totem und Tabu* and then inverts is not so much its anthropological material but rather the psychological mechanisms it describes. Like Erdheim, Marquard interprets *Totem und Tabu* in purely functionalistic terms, which makes questions such as whether there really was a primal horde effectively irrelevant.

The real problem with Marquard's ideas, it seems to me, lies elsewhere. Marquard neglects the fact that the German student revolution, rather than being an isolated national event, was part of a series of student protests in various countries, each with a history of its own. The theory of deferred disobedience may be applicable to Germany, to Italy, to France perhaps, but it has little explanatory power when it comes to the United States or Great Britain. Besides, many of the students' concerns were entirely legitimate. The war in Vietnam and, on a more modest scale, the highly authoritarian German university system were genuine wrongs; to criticize them was more than to discharge a mental need for revolt and direct it "against what happened to be there at the time: against . . . conditions that were democratic, liberal, and eminently worth preserving."[34]

Of course, this criticism does not invalidate Marquard's ideas. Marquard identifies *one* motivational force behind the German student revolution. The fact that there are other forces too only confirms Freud's theory of overdetermination. In other words, although Marquard himself views the German student revolution exclusively in terms of deferred disobedience, it is possible for a less reductive approach to incorporate his ideas into a larger framework that offers both a more comprehensive explanation and a more nuanced assessment.

Both Mario Erdheim and Odo Marquard use psychoanalysis to interpret contemporary social phenomena. But what does Freud himself have to say about modern society? To answer this question in full is impossible within the limited scope of this book. I shall therefore concentrate on a number of key insights that illustrate once more the critical nature of Freudian psychoanalysis. My starting-point will be Freud's *Zeitgemäßes über Krieg und Tod* (Thoughts for the Times on War and Death, 1915).

Man's Cultural Self-Deception

The word *Zeitgemäßes* literally means "that which is in keeping with the time." When in 1915, one year after the outbreak of the First World War, Freud published the long essay *Zeitgemäßes über Krieg und Tod,* he aimed to provide precisely that. He addressed people's questions about the war, about its causes, the extent to which it was or was not unavoidable, and its shockingly cruel nature. His answers were anything but uncontroversial.

The focal point of the essay is the disillusionment caused by the First World War. "We cannot but feel that no event has ever destroyed so much that is precious in the common possessions of humanity, confused so many of the clearest intelligences, or so thoroughly debased what is highest."[35] Whence, Freud asks, does this disillusionment come? His answer is that people did not expect a war, or at least not this kind of war. Armed conflicts, people told themselves, will continue to exist between underdeveloped nations, and between underdeveloped and developed nations, but not between developed nations, not between civilized *Kulturnationen*. Of course, even within those there are antisocial groups and individuals, but they constitute a minority. The state, people thought, will prevent or at least contain any antisocial behavior. And if a war did somehow come about, it would be "a chivalrous passage of arms,"[36] characterized by immunity for the wounded and the medical services, consideration for women and children, and respect for international law. But when the war came, there was nothing chivalrous about it. Bloodier and deadlier than any previous war, it completely ignored the rights of noncombatants and disregarded all international agreements, shattering people's hopes and convictions and causing widespread disillusionment.

After this straightforward start, Freud subjects the disillusionment brought about by the war to a closer, more controversial analysis. The disillusionment that people feel, he says, is not really justified, because it is based upon a false premise, the idea that the developed nations have reached a higher moral plane than the underdeveloped nations. Their members' primitive tendencies are wrongly supposed to have by and large been eradicated and replaced by good ones. Here Freud expounds the key thesis of the essay, a thesis which we have already come across in part 1 but which deserves to be quoted in full because it is central both to *Zeitgemäßes über Krieg und Tod* and to Freudian psychoanalysis as a whole. There is, Freud says,

> no such thing as "eradicating" evil. Psychological — or, more strictly speaking, psychoanalytic — investigation shows instead that the deepest essence of human nature consists of instinctual impulses [*Triebregungen*] which are of an elementary nature, which are similar in all men and which aim at the satisfaction of certain primal needs. These impulses in themselves are neither good nor bad. We classify them and their expressions in that way, according to their relation to the needs and demands of the human community. . . . These primitive impulses undergo a lengthy process of development before they are allowed to become active in the adult. They are inhibited, directed towards other aims and fields, become commingled, alter their objects, and are to some extent turned back upon their possessor. Reaction-formations against certain instincts [*Triebe*] take the deceptive form of a change in their content, as though egoism had changed into altruism, or cruelty into pity. These reaction-formations are facilitated by the circumstance that some instinctual impulses make their appearance almost from the first in pairs of opposites — a very remarkable phenomenon . . . which is termed "ambivalence of feeling."[37]

Man's primitive tendencies do not disappear through this process, because

> the development of the mind shows a peculiarity which is present in no other developmental process. When a village grows into a town or a child into a man, the village and the child become lost in the town and the man. Memory alone can trace the old features in the new picture; and in fact the old materials or forms have been got rid of and replaced by new ones. It is otherwise with the development of the mind. Here one can describe the state of affairs . . . only by saying that in this case every earlier stage of development persists alongside the later stage which has arisen from it; here succession also involves co-existence. . . . The earlier mental state may not have manifested itself for years, but none the less it is so far present that it may at any time again become the mode of expression of the forces in the mind, and indeed the only one, as though all later developments had been annulled or undone.[38]

People's shock and bewilderment at the horrors of the First World War are therefore strictly speaking naïve, man's unconscious wishful impulses being imperishable. Judged by them even "we ourselves are, like primaeval man, a gang of murderers."[39]

Against this backdrop, Freud examines three characteristics usually deemed typical of civilized man: his rational faculties, his altruistic inclinations, and his high moral standards.

One of the most striking features of the war was the apparent transformation of so many rational people into rabid warmongers. But we should not deceive ourselves, Freud says. Man is not the rational agent he thinks he is. Rather, it follows from the imperishable nature of the unconscious that man's intelligence and reason are neither the strongest forces operative in him nor even independent ones. The unconscious is a process which is always active and which all too often manages to force conscious motivations into its service. However important intelligence and reason may be, we cannot overlook their dependence on more primitive impulses: what man consciously and with complete sincerity tells himself is rational is all too frequently merely the manifestation of what he unconsciously desires.

Not only man's rational faculties, but also his feelings are elements of a more comprehensive mental life that for the most part is unknown to him. This is another reason why, contrary to what they like to believe, the members of the *Kulturnationen* have not risen above those of the other nations. Instead of having replaced their selfish urges, their altruistic inclinations constitute a reaction against them; they are a civilized way of dealing with a selfishness that is still present and that is just as powerful as before. The altruism of civilized man is thus not to be taken at face value, bound up as it is with negative tendencies that, though neither visible to others nor accessible to introspection, are there all the same. What makes the situation even more complex is that the altruistic reaction to selfish inclinations can take two entirely different forms. First, altruism can be put into the service of selfishness. By helping someone in need, for instance, we may satisfy our desire to feel superior and in control. Wars also exemplify this mechanism. A soldier is in a perfect position to obey the demands of the community, and thus be altruistic, by acting out aggressive feelings, acquiring possessions that belong to others, and so on. Second, instead of going along, as it were, with selfish inclinations, the altruistic reaction can do the exact opposite and block their path. As we saw in chapter 4, this is known as *Reaktionsbildung,* reaction-formation: the mind prevents selfish urges from manifesting themselves by fiercely pursuing their opposite, like a man trying to prevent an outburst of rage by overly correct behavior. It is therefore not surprising to find that

> the pre-existence of strong "bad" impulses in infancy is often the actual condition for an unmistakable inclination towards "good" in the adult. Those who as children have been the most pronounced egoists may well become the most helpful and self-sacrificing members of the community; most of our sentimentalists, friends of humanity and protectors of animals have evolved from little sadists and animal-tormentors.[40]

But whichever form a reaction against selfish urges takes, it does not eliminate them. Even though outwardly more altruistic, in his unconscious mind civilized man is just as primitive as his forebears.

Finally, let us turn to the remaining characteristic of civilized man, his high moral standards. Human beings, Freud writes, are induced to behave socially, first by their need to be loved and accepted by others (no one can survive without being part of a community) and second by their upbringing and education, which reward "good" actions and punish "bad" ones. It is for this reason that they start internalizing the moral standards of the community, thus developing a conscience. From this perspective, the sudden decline in moral standards during the First World War is hardly surprising. For "our conscience is not the inflexible judge that ethical teachers declare it, but in its origin is 'social anxiety' and nothing else."[41] The moment the community stops raising objections, there is more often than not "an end, too, to the suppression of evil passions, and men perpetrate deeds of cruelty, fraud, treachery and barbarity so incompatible with their level of civilization that one would have thought them impossible."[42]

To conclude, the developed nations may be more civilized than the underdeveloped ones (having a more elaborate legal system, less cruel forms of punishment, more charities, and so forth) but their members still have the same urges that have always been common to man. In contrast, then, to those cultural critics who, in the tradition of Jean-Jacques Rousseau, perceive man as essentially good and culture as a perverting influence, Freud has both a more pessimistic view of man and a more optimistic view of culture. Man in his original state, he asserts, is driven by antisocial urges that can only be contained through the renunciations and surrogate-satisfactions that society and culture require.

This does not mean, however, that Freud's position is uncritical. Quite the reverse. Precisely because psychoanalysis deals with society and culture in terms of their functional relevance, it is just as far removed from a self-congratulatory glorification of man's cultural achievements as it is from cultural pessimism à la Rousseau. Indeed, as we saw in chapter 3, the link between cultural phenomena and man's unconscious drives implies a fundamental skepticism towards any view of culture as the grand creation of autonomous individuals. What man considers to be his highest achievement is in reality, to take up the phrase I used toward the end of chapter 3, *the by-product of an unconscious survival strategy.* To look at society and culture from a psychoanalytic perspective is therefore also to expose man's cultural self-deception, his misunderstanding of his own achievements. And as this self-deception is itself a cultural phenomenon — it is to be found not just in individuals but also in the media, politics, science, and so on — the psychoanalytic study of culture is inevitably a critical one.

These reflections make it clear that the psychoanalytic theory of culture is not ahistorical, as so many critics of Freud have claimed. Freud, these critics say, views culture as a system of repressions and surrogate-satisfactions but he does so in general terms only. For him, man is a being whose essential antisocial drives can never be eradicated and who can therefore survive and coexist with others only in a community that suppresses and redirects these drives, so that there will always be a tension between man and culture. But, so the criticism goes, such a general "psychobiological" theory leaves no room for a critical assessment of historically specific phenomena.

This criticism is too simple. It is true that in Freud's view any society is of necessity repressive, but the factors that lead to repression and surrogate-satisfaction are historically variable. The institutions, laws, rules, and the like that prevent people from acting out their drives are concrete social phenomena; and people's consciences, which urge them to conform to the demands of the community, have their origins in concrete social values and expectations. This automatically raises the question as to the relative merits and demerits of these different factors. "The essential question," Freud writes in *Die Zukunft einer Illusion* (The Future of an Illusion, 1927), "is whether and to what extent it is possible to lessen the burden of the instinctual sacrifices [*Triebopfer*] imposed on men, to reconcile men to those which must necessarily remain and to provide a compensation for them."[43] In other words, the psychoanalytic approach draws attention, not simply to a general tension between man's drives and society's demands, but to the historically specific conditions that lead to drive-renunciation, drive-redirection, or drive-satisfaction.

As a critical theory of society and culture, psychoanalysis is apt to cause far more discomfort than as a branch of the medical sciences. As a medical science, psychoanalysis focuses on abnormal behavior; the unconscious impulses it seeks to uncover are characteristic of an abnormal state of mind. As a form of social critique, by contrast, psychoanalysis is about *normal* behavior; the unconscious impulses it exposes are characteristic of *us*. In the remaining pages of this book, I wish to illustrate the essential difference between these two types of psychoanalysis by examining the case of the Belgian pedophile Marc Dutroux and the public reactions to it.

Two Types of Psychoanalysis

In 1996, Marc Dutroux was driven in an armored police car to the courthouse in the Belgian town of Neufchâteau to stand trial for the abduction, sexual abuse, and murder of four girls aged between eight and nineteen and the abduction and sexual abuse of two other young girls. An angry crowd was waiting for him, hurling abuses at the "perverted swine," and demanding his immediate death or castration. Had Dutroux not been escorted by armed police, the demonstrators would undoubtedly have taken the law into their own hands, and the trial would have been over before it had even begun.

What do we see when we look at these events from the perspective of psychoanalysis? If we understand psychoanalysis purely as a medical science, the answer is straightforward enough. We see a homicidal pedophile on one side, a society which is appalled by his crimes and rightfully seeks to protect itself on the other. Dutroux is mentally ill and in need of treatment; society, as long as it has not cured him, needs to keep him securely separated from the rest of the population. From the perspective of psychoanalysis as a critical theory of society and culture, the answer is less straightforward. This type of psychoanalysis widens the focus, examining as it does not just deviant behavior but *all* forms of behavior. Its aim is not simply to cure mentally ill people but to render visible the interplay of conscious and unconscious drives in the ill *and* the healthy. From this perspective, the dichotomy of society on the one hand and Dutroux on the other — of *us* and *him* — cannot be upheld. It is no longer a case of one individual needing psychoanalytic examination, as against a society that raises no matters of psychoanalytic concern. Now the behavior of all people concerned is a psychoanalytic issue.

This does not mean that Dutroux ceases to be a dangerous sex-offender, or that there is no longer any need to lock him away and subject him to treatment, or that society loses the right to do so. From the point of view of psychoanalysis as a form of social critique, too, there remains a crucial difference between those who commit sex-crimes and those who do not. After all, what distinguishes people from one another, according to Freud, is not that they have different primitive drives but that they deal with the same primitive drives in different ways. Or, to put it in a less misleading manner, what distinguishes people from one another is the different outlets their drives manage to find. And the criminal outlet of Dutroux's drives clearly sets him apart from others.

But what about those others? What insights does psychoanalysis provide when it widens the focus and examines the events surrounding Dutroux's arrest and trial?

Perhaps the most striking feature of the Dutroux case is the public reactions it generated. For months on end, Belgium and indeed Europe were in the grip of *l'affaire Dutroux*. An endless stream of newspaper and magazine articles as well as radio and television features covered every aspect of the case, from Dutroux's personal background to the minutiae of the police investigation. But it was not only the media that threw themselves upon Dutroux's crimes. The general public also became engaged on a massive scale. The victims' parents were inundated with expressions of sympathy; there were vigils and silent marches; citizens' action groups sprang up like mushrooms. Dutroux, it seemed, had become evil incarnate.

Up to a point, these reactions are understandable. Pedophilia is a genuine social problem, and Dutroux's crimes were of a particularly gruesome nature. Moreover, there was some indication that Dutroux was part of an international pedophile ring comprising, among others, politicians and high-ranking civil servants who were now trying to cover up their involvement. These allegations were never substantiated but obviously attracted attention. Yet all this explains neither the scale of public engagement nor the vehemence of the reactions. In particular, what remains unexplained is the way people looked upon Dutroux: as if he were a kind of demon rather than simply a vicious criminal.

What, then, are we to make of the overwhelming interest stirred up by Dutroux's crimes? And what, in particular, are we to make of the almost hysterical fear Dutroux inspired? A hint can be found when we recall Ernest Jones's analysis of Hamlet's behavior towards his mother. On the surface, Hamlet is appalled at his mother's sexual relationship with her brother-in-law. He vehemently reproaches her for her wantonness and in effect likens her to a prostitute. But, as we saw, it is precisely this reaction that points to his repressed desire for his mother. Hamlet's excessive outward disgust betrays his powerful inward fascination; his raging and shouting constitute an unconscious strategy to drown out the seductive voice of his id. The parallel with the reactions to Dutroux's behavior is unmistakable. They, too, are disproportionately emotional. They, too, combine vehement rejection with a penchant for graphic detail, moral indignation with prying curiosity, and disgust with active engagement. It would appear, then, that Dutroux's critics are actually more than a little fascinated with his crimes.

From the standpoint of conventional morality, such a suggestion must appear positively blasphemous. Is it not right and proper to be repelled and frightened by sex-crimes? Surely the people who denounced Dutroux did so because they found his actions sickening? How can one conclude from their *repulsion* that they are *attracted* to his crimes? From a Freudian perspective, however, such "perverse" logic is simply the reflection of psychological reality. All mental life is ambivalent, and the force with which conscious feelings are experienced, expressed, or defended is as a rule commensurate with the force of their unconscious opposite. Moreover, Freud has shown that lustful and aggressive drives are not restricted to deviants or perverts but are common to all humanity and, furthermore, that more often than not they take as their object those who are nearest and dearest to us or those who are the most vulnerable. All this suggests that the extreme nature of the reactions to

Dutroux results from the psychological process we have come to know as *reaction-formation;* in other words, that it is the outcome of an unconscious strategy to transform a mixture of abhorrence and fascination into pure abhorrence.

This approach also helps us to understand the media attention the case generated. Viewed psychoanalytically, the excessive production and consumption of articles, editorials, photo features, news broadcasts, and documentaries are to be interpreted as forms of *sublimation*. They are unconscious attempts to divert the energy of primitive, antisocial drives into socially acceptable activities. They do so in such a way as to satisfy both the id's desire for sexual perversity and the superego's desire for moral purity. Not only do they offer people the opportunity to experience the thrill of the forbidden but they also enable them to share in the general atmosphere of condemnation. The relief provided consists in the satisfaction of mental ambivalence. A similar psychological mechanism can be detected in the aggression displayed by the crowd waiting in front of the courthouse. The verbal and attempted physical abuse of Dutroux represent, I would suggest, a form of *surrogate satisfaction:* the primitive impulses stirred up by Dutroux's crimes but rejected by the superego find vent by attaching themselves to a socially acceptable surrogate object, Dutroux himself.

But what about the almost hysterical fear inspired by Dutroux? Why were people so afraid of him even after he had been caught and imprisoned? Psychoanalysis distinguishes between three types of fear or anxiety: realistic anxiety, moral anxiety, and neurotic anxiety. Realistic anxiety has its source in the outside world, in a wild animal crossing one's path, a burglar trying to get in, and so on. Moral anxiety has its source in the norms and values one has internalized; it is fear of being punished by the superego. For instance, a masturbating child may be anxious both because he is afraid that his parents might find out (realistic anxiety) and because he feels guilty (moral anxiety). Often, realistic anxiety and moral anxiety interact to a point where it is no longer possible to determine where the one ends and the other begins. A good example is the fear felt by the protagonist of Edgar Allan Poe's "The Tell-Tale Heart." Neurotic anxiety, finally, is fear of the object-choice of the id. Phobias, such as an irrational fear of heights, can often be explained in this way. Standing on the edge of a cliff, albeit behind a solid fence, many people take fright because they cannot help thinking what would happen if they jumped. This type of anxiety is frequently heightened by moral anxiety. Thus, a married man may be anxious about going on a business trip with his attractive secretary because he is afraid that he might be unable to control his sexual urges, and this anxiety may then be increased by moral scruples.

We are now able to identify the psychological structure of the fear of Dutroux. One of the most common defense mechanisms of the unconscious mind is the use of *projection* to transform moral or neurotic anxiety into realistic anxiety. Unconscious lustful, aggressive desires are detached from oneself and ascribed to someone else and thus ejected, as it were, from the mind into the outside world. As a result, the threat becomes an external one: the anxiety is objectified.[44] This, it seems to me, is what happened in the case of Dutroux. For fear that their repressed id-desires might return — a fear increased by pressure from the superego — people externalized these desires and projected them onto Dutroux. When looking at Dutroux, they no longer saw a dangerous criminal but the inner demon they had exorcised. They saw the terrifying face of their own id.

My analysis of the Dutroux case has served to illustrate the distinction between the critical and the medical applications of psychoanalysis. I do not mean to imply that psychoanalysis cannot or should not be applied as a medical science. Freud himself used psychoanalysis for therapeutic purposes, often very successfully. As other analysts since have also obtained good results, it would be absurd to argue for an exclusively critical use of Freud's ideas. Besides, the distinction between the two types of psychoanalysis is not absolute. Both seek to render visible what people do not know, indeed do not want to know, about themselves. By peeling away the layers of self-deception that cover the interplay of consciousness and unconsciousness, both aim to provide people with a more realistic picture of themselves and the world. Still, a crucial difference remains: whereas therapeutic psychoanalysis deals with actions or feelings that constitute a problem for the individual or society, critical psychoanalysis examines what is generally perceived to be unproblematic. It turns its suspicious gaze on the very things that are considered normal or morally unambiguous, that are celebrated as expressions of what is noblest and highest in man, or are neglected as being trivial and irrelevant. The importance that Freud himself attached to this critical approach is apparent from his work on such phenomena as social taboos, art and literature, and faulty actions.

Extending as it does beyond the realm of the medico-psychological, psychoanalysis questions society's self-image. In this respect, Freud's ideas resemble those of Karl Marx (1818–1883), that other great *master of suspicion,* to use Paul Ricoeur's phrase. According to Marx, political, moral, religious, esthetic, and other theories and doctrines (as well as the actions based on them) are determined by deeper-lying socio-economic developments: they reflect socio-economic conflicts and constitute a pseudo-solution to them. Religious belief, for example, is for Marx the reflection of an imperfect world, a world in which the majority of the people cannot realize their full potential. People turn to religion because religion helps them to come to terms with their misery by justifying the existing order as God-given and holding out the promise of happiness in the hereafter. So people accept the world as it is — and the conflict between the needs they have and the opportunities society offers (a conflict that, according to Marxism, is in reality based on an unjust system of economic production and distribution) is "solved." Religion for Marx is thus not a confidence trick perpetrated by the ruling classes on the less well-off in order to keep them quiet, but a kind of drug to which both the haves and the have-nots resort so as not to feel the pain of social injustice. (That is why Marx says that religion is the opium *of* the people and not, as he is often misquoted, *for* the people.) This process works because people do not see through it. They think they simply believe in God, not knowing — nor wanting to know — that their belief is groundless and merely constitutes an escape from, and a justification of, their misery. Religion is one of the means by which the individual and society deceive themselves about the true state of affairs. To use a phrase of Marx's collaborator Friedrich Engels (1820–1895), it is a form of *false consciousness.*

The task that Marxist analysis sets itself is to trace back such forms of false consciousness to their socio-economic roots. Its aim is to lay bare the social forces behind moral, religious, esthetic, and other beliefs and convictions, which people themselves view as resulting from free choice. So Marxist analysis does not simply focus on these beliefs and convictions as such; it does not simply seek to show that they are inconsistent or unconvincingly argued. Rather, it analyzes them as elements of the total-ity of social life. It seeks to uncover their dependence on a social struc-ture that is not immediately visible precisely because it is obscured by these theories and doctrines. Thus, to take up our example again, people do not see that it is the economic system that is at the root of their mis-ery, because religion tells them that their misery is God's will.

The similarities with psychoanalysis are obvious. Psychoanalysis, too, is fundamentally suspicious of people's beliefs and convictions, and of people's view that their beliefs and convictions are wholly of their own making. Psychoanalysis, too, considers phenomena such as morality, religion, and esthetics (and the behavior based on them) to be depend-ent on forces of which people themselves are unaware. And, again like Marxist analysis, psychoanalysis regards these forms of false consciousness both as reflections of deeper-lying conflicts and as attempts to solve them. The excessive moral indignation and fear displayed towards Marc Dutroux, for instance, turned out to be expressive of both an uncon-scious conflict between id-desires and superego-desires, and of a way to reconcile them. In short, both Marx and Freud expose the seemingly innocuous and respectable as means by which the individual and society unknowingly cover up their imperfections.

This does not mean that there are no important differences between psychoanalysis and Marxist analysis. First, according to Freud false con-sciousness, rather than having its foundation in socio-economic condi-tions, results from a conflict between antisocial drives and social demands. Of course, such conflicts may be related to socio-economic issues. The extent to which women have access to the labor-market, for example, obviously affects their psychosexual development. But the conflicts that psychoanalysis identifies are *not always* and *not necessarily* ultimately determined by the way the production and distribution of goods are organized. Second, whereas for Marx the various forms of false consciousness constitute merely a pseudo-solution to the problems of the individual and society, Freud takes a more positive view of these socio-psychological defense mechanisms. To be sure, for Freud, too, reaction-formation, sublimation, projection, and so on are shields against an unpleasant reality, devices with which people fend off unwanted prob-lems. But for him they are more than that. He views them as in many cases useful compromises, ways in which people potentially not just evade the contradictions they are faced with but actually manage to reconcile them. Freud is far more skeptical than Marx about the possibility of perfect solutions.

This brings us to the third and last key difference between psychoanalysis and Marxist analysis. For Marx, true happiness presupposes the elimination of all false consciousness, which in its turn presupposes the revolutionary overhaul of the socio-economic structure of society. Marxism therefore aims not simply to analyze the world but to change it. Freud, by contrast, does not believe in such radical solutions. In his view, finding a balance between antisocial drives and social demands will always be a matter of muddling through. The aim of psychoanalysis is correspondingly modest: to help people develop a more realistic picture of themselves and the world so that, perhaps, with increased self-knowledge the more pernicious forms of false consciousness might be avoided.

Yet despite these fundamental differences, Freud's theory has the same thrust as that of Marx: it aims not simply to criticize what people believe and do but to analyze their beliefs and actions as the outward manifestation of a more comprehensive reality that for the most part remains unknown to them. It seeks to lay bare the multilayered nature of reality, its fundamental complexity and ambiguity. And in doing so it subverts the reductive classifications with which people preserve the safe one-dimensionality of their world-view.

How attractive such classifications are can be seen even from my own analysis of the case of Marc Dutroux. On one level, this analysis questioned the reassuring dichotomy of Dutroux and society by demonstrating that Dutroux and his critics were driven by essentially similar desires. On another level, however, it merely reproduced this dichotomy in a different form. It focused on Dutroux's critics as other people, as *them* rather than *us,* and left things at that. The analysis was broken off before it could become genuinely uncomfortable. Pursued to the end, it would have resulted in an examination of the psychological function of the analysis itself. Is my analysis of the behavior of Dutroux and his critics perhaps also a form of sublimation? To what extent is my criticism of Dutroux's critics itself a form of projection? Might my detached approach not be an instance of reaction-formation? And what about you, the reader? Might not the *reading* of all this satisfy certain unconscious desires, too? To ask such questions is not retrospectively to devalue the analysis. We know that psychoanalytic investigations can fulfill projective, sublimatory, or other psychological functions and yet provide important insights; Freud's own *Totem und Tabu* is a case in point. The psycho-analytic law of overdetermination also applies to psychoanalysis itself. But the questions do remind us that, as far as Freudian theory is concerned, there can be no simple *us* versus *them,* and no criticism without self-criticism. In the words of Bernd Nitzschke:

> Freud knew that the accusatory finger pointed at another person is al-ways accompanied by three further fingers pointing back towards the accuser. His true object of study and focus of interest was never other people, but always *ourselves.*[45]

Notes

[1] A. L. Kroeber, "Totem and Taboo in Retrospect" [1939], in *The Nature of Culture* (Chicago: U of Chicago P, 1952), 306.

[2] Sigmund Freud, *The Origins of Religion,* trans. James Strachey, ed. Albert Dickson, vol. 13 of *The Penguin Freud Library,* ed. Angela Richards and Albert Dickson (Harmondsworth: Penguin, 1990), 54–55.

[3] Freud, *Origins of Religion,* 71.

[4] Freud, *Origins of Religion,* 71; translation modified.

[5] Freud, *Origins of Religion,* 165.

[6] Freud, *Origins of Religion,* 81.

[7] Freud, *Origins of Religion,* 81–82.

[8] According to Freud, a remnant of this belief — that the dead drag the living in their train, that the dead kill — can be found in the image of death as a skeleton with scythe. Death, this image implies, is itself dead (Freud, *Origins of Religion,* 114–15; with reference to Rudolf Kleinpaul).

[9] Freud, *Origins of Religion,* 119.

[10] The German phrase is *nachträglicher Gehorsam,* which in older translations is rendered by "subsequent obedience."

[11] Freud, *Origins of Religion,* 204–5.

[12] Freud, *Origins of Religion,* 206.

[13] Freud, *Origins of Religion,* 219.

[14] Freud, *Origins of Religion,* 220–21.

[15] Freud, *Origins of Religion*, 221; translation modified.

[16] Here, I follow Mario Erdheim, "Einleitung," in Sigmund Freud, *Totem und Tabu. Einige Übereinstimmungen im Seelenleben der Wilden und der Neurotiker* (Frankfurt am Main: Fischer, 1995), 21–23.

[17] Freud, *Totem und Tabu*, 23.

[18] The following account is based on Manfred Dierks, "Thomas Mann und die Tiefenpsychologie," in Helmut Koopmann, ed., *Thomas-Mann-Handbuch*, 2nd ed. (Stuttgart: Kröner, 1995), 284–300; see also Erdheim, "Einleitung," 9–11.

[19] Thomas Mann, *Freud und die Psychoanalyse. Reden, Briefe, Notizen, Betrachtungen*, ed. Bernd Urban (Frankfurt am Main: Fischer, 1991), 122.

[20] Mann, *Freud und die Psychoanalyse. Reden, Briefe, Notizen, Betrachtungen*, 133.

[21] See Erdheim, "Einleitung," 10.

[22] Ernst Jünger, *Der Kampf als inneres Erlebnis*, 6th ed. (Berlin: Mittler, 1936), 7–8; quoted in Erdheim, "Einleitung," 10–11.

[23] Erdheim, "Einleitung."

[24] Freud, *Origins of Religion*, 84.

[25] Freud, *Origins of Religion*, 81.

[26] Of course, Erdheim's explanation does not exclude, and is undoubtedly not meant to exclude, other explanations of the taboos attached to the way Germany deals with its past. As with other phenomena, taboos tend to be overdetermined.

[27] Odo Marquard, "Farewell to Matters of Principle. (Another Autobiographical Introduction)," in *Farewell to Matters of Principle: Philosophical Studies*, trans. Robert M. Wallace et al. (New York/Oxford: Oxford UP, 1989).

[28] Marquard, "Farewell to Matters of Principle," 10.

[29] In *Auf dem Weg zur vaterlosen Gesellschaft* (Society without the Father, 1963), Alexander Mitscherlich puts forward the thesis that in modern society the main formative influence on the child is no longer the father or the patriarchal family, but the all-pervasive ideology of industrial capitalism. By analogy, Marquard argues that during National Socialism the father was replaced by Hitler and Hitlerite ideology.

[30] Marquard, "Farewell to Matters of Principle," 8–9; translation modified.

[31] Marquard, "Farewell to Matters of Principle," 10.

[32] Marquard, "Farewell to Matters of Principle," 10.

[33] Marquard, "Farewell to Matters of Principle," 12.

[34] Marquard, "Farewell to Matters of Principle," 9.

[35] Sigmund Freud, *Civilization, Society and Religion*, trans. James Strachey, ed. Albert Dickson, vol. 12 of *The Penguin Freud Library*, ed. Angela Richards and Albert Dickson (Harmondsworth: Penguin, 1990), 61.

[36] Freud, *Civilization, Society and Religion*, 64.

[37] Freud, *Civilization, Society and Religion,* 68.

[38] Freud, *Civilization, Society and Religion,* 73.

[39] Freud, *Civilization, Society and Religion,* 86.

[40] Freud, *Civilization, Society and Religion,* 69; translation modified.

[41] Freud, *Civilization, Society and Religion,* 66–67.

[42] Freud, *Civilization, Society and Religion,* 67.

[43] Freud, *Civilization, Society and Religion,* 186; see also Alfred Lorenzer and Bernard Görlich, "Einleitung," in Sigmund Freud, *Das Unbehagen in der Kultur und andere kulturtheoretische Schriften* (Frankfurt am Main: Fischer, 1997), 15.

[44] See Freud's analysis of the "primitive" fear of the dead discussed in the section on *"Totem and Taboo* I" at the beginning of this chapter.

[45] Bernd Nitzschke, *Wir und der Tod. Essays über Sigmund Freuds Leben und Werk* (Göttingen: Vandenhoeck & Ruprecht, 1996), 52.

Bibliography

BESIDES WORKS REFERRED TO in the text, this bibliography includes a selection of studies on psychoanalysis and psychoanalytic literary and cultural criticism that I found particularly useful. They may help the reader in further exploring the issues discussed in this book.

Beland, Hermann. "Nachwort." In Sigmund Freud, *Die Traumdeutung,* 629–54. Frankfurt am Main: Fischer, 1991.

Bernfeld, Siegfried, and Suzanne Bernfeld. *Bausteine der Freud-Biographik.* Trans. and ed. Ilse Grubrich-Simitis. Frankfurt am Main: Suhrkamp, 1988.

Bettelheim, Bruno. *Freud and Man's Soul.* London: Chatto & Windus/The Hogarth Press, 1983.

———. *The Uses of Enchantment: The Meaning and Importance of Fairy Tales.* 1976. Reprint, Harmondsworth: Penguin, 1991.

Bonaparte, Marie. *The Life and Works of Edgar Allan Poe: A Psycho-Analytic Interpretation.* Trans. John Rodker. Foreword by Sigmund Freud. London: Imago, 1949 (first published in French 1933).

Brome, Vincent. *Freud and His Disciples.* London: House of Stratus, 2001.

Brown, J. A. C. *Freud and the Post-Freudians.* Rev. ed. Harmondsworth: Penguin, 1964.

Clark, Ronald W. *Freud: The Man and the Cause.* New York: Random House, 1980.

Costigan, Giovanni. *Sigmund Freud: A Short Biography.* London: Robert Hale, 1967.

Dierks, Manfred. "Thomas Mann und die Tiefenpsychologie." In *Thomas-Mann-Handbuch,* ed. Helmut Koopmann, 284–300. 2nd ed. Stuttgart: Kröner, 1995.

Eissler, K. R. *Goethe: A Psychoanalytic Study 1775–1786.* Detroit: Wayne State UP, 1963.

Ellenberger, Henri F. *The Discovery of the Unconscious: The History and Evolution of Dynamic Psychiatry.* 1970. Reprint, London: Fontana, 1994.

Ellmann, Maud, ed. *Psychoanalytic Literary Criticism*. London/New York: Longman, 1994.

Erdheim, Mario. *Die gesellschaftliche Produktion von Unbewußtheit. Eine Einführung in den ethnopsychoanalytischen Prozeß*. Frankfurt am Main: Suhrkamp, 1982.

———. *Psychoanalyse und Unbewußtheit in der Kultur. Aufsätze 1980–1987*. 3rd ed. Frankfurt am Main: Suhrkamp, 1994.

———. "Einleitung." In Sigmund Freud, *Totem und Tabu. Einige Übereinstimmungen im Seelenleben der Wilden und der Neurotiker*, 7–42. Frankfurt am Main: Fischer, 1995.

Ferris, Paul. *Dr Freud: A Life*. London: Sinclair Stevenson, 1997.

Fischer, Jens Malte, ed. *Psychoanalytische Literaturinterpretation. Aufsätze aus "Imago. Zeitschrift für Anwendung der Psychoanalyse auf die Geisteswissenschaften" (1912–1937)*. Deutsche Texte 54. Munich and Tübingen: dtv and Niemeyer, 1980.

Forster, Leonard, ed. *The Penguin Book of German Verse*. Rev. ed. Harmondsworth: Penguin, 1959.

Fraiberg, Louis. *Psychoanalysis & American Literary Criticism*. Detroit: Wayne State UP, 1960.

Freud, Ernst, Lucie Freud, and Ilse Grubrich-Simitis. *Sigmund Freud: His Life in Pictures and Words*. Trans. Christine Trollope. New York/London: W. W. Norton, 1985 (first published in German 1976).

Freud, Sigmund. *The Penguin Freud Library*. Ed. Angela Richards and Albert Dickson. 15 vols. Harmondsworth: Penguin, 1990–1993. (Reprint of *The Pelican Freud Library*, 1973–1986.)

Vol. 1: *Introductory Lectures on Psychoanalysis*. Trans. James Strachey. Ed. James Strachey and Angela Richards. 1973, 1991.

Vol. 2: *New Introductory Lectures on Psychoanalysis*. Trans. James Strachey. Ed. James Strachey with the assistance of Angela Richards. 1973, 1991.

Vol. 3: *Studies on Hysteria*. Trans. James and Alix Strachey. Ed. Angela Richards. 1974, 1991.

Vol. 4: *The Interpretation of Dreams*. Trans. James Strachey. Ed. Angela Richards. 1976, 1991.

Vol. 5: *The Psychopathology of Everyday Life*. Trans. Alan Tyson. Ed. Angela Richards. 1975, 1991.

Vol. 6: *Jokes and Their Relation to the Unconscious.* Trans. James Strachey. Ed. Angela Richards. 1976, 1991.

Vol. 7: *On Sexuality.* Trans. James Strachey. Ed. Angela Richards. 1977, 1991.

Vol. 8: *Case Histories I.* Trans. Alix and James Strachey. Ed. Angela Richards. 1977, 1990.

Vol. 9: *Case Histories II.* Trans. James Strachey. Ed. Angela Richards. 1979, 1991.

Vol. 10: *On Psychopathology.* Trans. James Strachey. Ed. Angela Richards. 1979, 1993.

Vol. 11: *On Metapsychology.* Trans. James Strachey. Ed. Angela Richards. 1984, 1991.

Vol. 12: *Civilization, Society and Religion.* Trans. James Strachey. Ed. Albert Dickson. 1985, 1991.

Vol. 13: *The Origins of Religion.* Trans. James Strachey. Ed. Albert Dickson. 1985, 1990.

Vol. 14: *Art and Literature.* Trans. James Strachey. Ed. Albert Dickson. 1985, 1990.

Vol. 15: *Historical and Expository Works on Psychoanalysis.* Trans. James Strachey. Ed. Albert Dickson. 1986, 1993.

————. *Two Short Accounts of Psycho-Analysis.* Ed. and trans. James Strachey. Harmondsworth: Penguin, 1977.

Galsworthy, John. *The Island Pharisees.* 1904. Reprint, London: Heinemann, 1927.

Gay, Peter. *Freud for Historians.* New York/Oxford: Oxford UP, 1985.

————. *Freud: A Life for Our Time.* New York/London: W. W. Norton, 1988.

————. *Reading Freud: Explorations and Entertainments.* New Haven/London: Yale UP, 1990.

Glaser, Hermann. *Sigmund Freuds Zwanzigstes Jahrhundert. Seelenbilder einer Epoche. Materialien und Analysen.* Frankfurt am Main: Fischer, 1979.

Gordon, David J. *Literary Art and the Unconscious.* Baton Rouge: Louisiana State UP, 1976.

Görlich, Bernard. *Die Wette mit Freud. Drei Studien zu Herbert Marcuse.* Frankfurt am Main: Nexus, 1991.

Görlich, Bernard, Alfred Lorenzer, and Alfred Schmidt. *Der Stachel Freud. Beiträge und Dokumente zur Kulturismuskritik. Mit Texten von Otto Fenichel, Th. W. Adorno, Max Horkheimer und Herbert Marcuse.* Frankfurt am Main: Suhrkamp, 1980.

Hall, Calvin S. *A Primer of Freudian Psychology.* New York: Mentor/New American Library, 1954.

Heine, Heinrich. *Historisch-kritische Gesamtausgabe der Werke.* Ed. Manfred Windfuhr. Hamburg: Hoffmann und Campe, 1973–.

Hoffman, Frederick J. *Freudianism and the Literary Mind.* 2nd rev. ed. Baton Rouge: Louisiana State UP, 1957.

Höhn, Gerhard. *Heine-Handbuch. Zeit, Person, Werk.* 2nd rev. ed. Stuttgart/Weimar: Metzler, 1997.

Holland, Norman N. *Psychoanalysis and Shakespeare.* New York/London/Toronto: McGraw-Hill, 1966.

———. *Poems in Persons: An Introduction to the Psychoanalysis of Literature.* New York: W. W. Norton, 1973.

———. *Holland's Guide to Psychoanalytic Psychology and Literature-and-Psychology.* New York and Oxford: Oxford UP, 1990.

Jones, Ernest. *What Is Psychoanalysis?* London: George Allen & Unwin, 1949.

———. *Sigmund Freud: Life and Work.* 3 vols. London: The Hogarth Press, 1953–1957.

———. *Hamlet and Oedipus.* 1949. Reprint, New York/London: W. W. Norton, 1976.

Kaplan, Morton, and Robert Kloss. *The Unspoken Motive: A Guide to Psychoanalytic Literary Criticism.* New York: The Free Press, 1973.

Kiell, Norman, ed. *Psychoanalysis, Psychology, and Literature: A Bibliography.* 2nd ed. Metuchen, NJ/London: The Scarecrow Press, 1982.

Kroeber, A. L. "Totem and Taboo: An Ethnologic Analysis" [1920]. In *The Nature of Culture,* 301–5, 422. Chicago: U of Chicago P, 1952.

———. "Totem and Taboo in Retrospect" [1939]. In *The Nature of Culture,* 306–9. Chicago: U of Chicago P, 1952.

Laplanche, J., and J.-B. Pontalis. *The Language of Psycho-Analysis.* Trans. Donald Nicholson-Smith, with an introduction by Daniel Lagache. London: Karnac and the Institute of Psycho-Analysis, 1988 (first published in French 1967).

Lesser, Simon O. *Fiction and the Unconscious.* With a preface by Ernest Jones. Chicago/London: U of Chicago P, 1957.

———. *The Whispered Meanings: Selected Essays of Simon O. Lesser.* Ed. Robert Sprich and Richard W. Noland. Amherst: U of Massachusetts P, 1977.

Lohmann, Hans-Martin. *Freud zur Einführung.* Zur Einführung 71. Hamburg: Junius, 1986.

———, ed. *Die Psychoanalyse auf der Couch.* Frankfurt am Main: Fischer, 1986.

———. *Alexander Mitscherlich.* Reinbek bei Hamburg: Rowohlt, 1987.

———. *Freud.* Reinbek bei Hamburg: Rowohlt, 1998.

Lorenzer, Alfred, and Bernard Görlich. "Einleitung." In Sigmund Freud, *Das Unbehagen in der Kultur und andere kulturtheoretische Schriften,* 7–28. Frankfurt am Main: Fischer, 1997.

Lütkehaus, Ludger, ed. *Tiefenphilosophie. Texte zur Entdeckung des Unbewußten vor Freud.* 1989. Reprint, Hamburg: Europäische Verlagsanstalt, 1995.

Manheim, Leonard, and Eleanor Manheim, ed. *Hidden Patterns: Studies in Psychoanalytic Literary Criticism.* New York: Macmillan, 1966.

Mann, Thomas. *Freud und die Psychoanalyse. Reden, Briefe, Notizen, Betrachtungen.* Ed. Bernd Urban. Frankfurt am Main: Fischer, 1991.

Mannoni, Octave. *Freud.* Reinbek bei Hamburg: Rowohlt, 1971.

Marquard, Odo. "Farewell to Matters of Principle. (Another Autobiographical Introduction)." In *Farewell to Matters of Principle: Philosophical Studies.* Trans. Robert M. Wallace with the assistance of Susan Bernstein and James I. Porter, 3–21. New York/Oxford: Oxford UP, 1989 (first published in German 1981).

Mentzos, Stavros. "Einleitung." In Josef Breuer and Sigmund Freud, *Studien über Hysterie,* 7–20. 4th ed. Frankfurt am Main: Fischer, 2000.

Mitscherlich, Alexander. *Society without the Father: A Contribution to Social Psychology.* Trans. Eric Mosbacher. London: Tavistock Publications, 1969 (first published in German 1963).

———. "Der Kampf um die Erinnerung. Psychoanalyse für fortgeschrittene Anfänger" [1975]. In *Gesammelte Schriften VIII: Psychoanalyse,* ed. Max Looser, 385–574. Frankfurt am Main: Suhrkamp, 1983.

Mollinger, Robert N. *Psychoanalysis and Literature: An Introduction.* Chicago: Nelson-Hall, 1981.

Morrison, Claudia C. *Freud and the Critic: The Early Use of Depth Psychology in Literary Criticism.* Chapel Hill: U of North Carolina P, 1968.

Neu, Jerome, ed. *The Cambridge Companion to Freud.* Cambridge: Cambridge UP, 1991.

Newton, Peter M. *Freud: From Youthful Dream to Mid-Life Crisis.* New York/London: Guilford, 1995.

Nitzschke, Bernd. *Wir und der Tod. Essays über Sigmund Freuds Leben und Werk.* Göttingen: Vandenhoeck & Ruprecht, 1996.

———. *Aufbruch nach Inner-Afrika. Essays über Sigmund Freud und die Wurzeln der Psychoanalyse.* Göttingen: Vandenhoeck & Ruprecht, 1998.

———. *Das Ich als Experiment. Essays über Sigmund Freud und die Psychoanalyse im 20. Jahrhundert.* Göttingen: Vandenhoeck & Ruprecht, 2000.

Phillips, William, ed. *Art and Psychoanalysis.* New York: Criterion Books, 1957.

Reh, Albert M. *Literatur und Psychologie.* Germanistische Lehrbuchsammlung 72. Berne/Frankfurt am Main/New York: Lang, 1986.

Reppen, Joseph, and Maurice Charney, eds. *The Psychoanalytic Study of Literature.* Hillsdale, NJ: The Analytic Press, 1985.

Richards, Barry. *Images of Freud: Cultural Responses to Psychoanalysis.* London: J. M. Dent & Sons, 1989.

Ruitenbeek, Hendrik M. *The Literary Imagination: Psychoanalysis and the Genius of the Writer.* Chicago: Quadrangle Books, 1965.

Schneider, Peter. *Sigmund Freud.* Munich: dtv, 1999.

Schönau, Walter. "Literarisches Lesen in psychoanalytischer Sicht." *Freiburger literaturpsychologische Gespräche* 4 (1985): 9–26.

———. *Einführung in die psychoanalytische Literaturwissenschaft.* Sammlung Metzler 259. Stuttgart: Metzler, 1991.

Shakespeare, William. *The Merchant of Venice.* Ed. John Russell Brown. The Arden Shakespeare. London: Methuen, 1961.

———. *Hamlet.* Ed. Harold Jenkins. The Arden Shakespeare. London: Methuen, 1982.

Spector, Jack J. *The Aesthetics of Freud.* New York: Praeger, 1972.

Speziale-Bagliacca, Roberto. *Sigmund Freud.* Trans. Petra Kaiser. Heidelberg: Spektrum der Wissenschaft, 2000.

Stafford-Clark, David. *What Freud Really Said*. 1965. Reprint, Harmondsworth: Penguin, 1992.

Steiner, Riccardo. "Einleitung." In Sigmund Freud, *Zur Psychopathologie des Alltagslebens. Über Vergessen, Versprechen, Vergreifen, Aberglaube und Irrtum*, 7–60. Frankfurt am Main: Fischer, 2000.

Storr, Anthony. *Freud: A Very Short Introduction*. 1989. Reprint, Oxford/New York: Oxford UP, 2001.

Sulloway, Frank J. *Freud, Biologist of the Mind: Beyond the Psychoanalytic Legend*. London: Burnett Books, 1979.

Urban, Bernd, ed. *Psychoanalyse und Literaturwissenschaft. Texte zur Geschichte ihrer Beziehungen*. Tübingen: Niemeyer, 1973.

Vice, Sue, ed. *Psychoanalytic Criticism: A Reader*. Cambridge: Polity Press, 1996.

von Matt, Peter. *Literaturwissenschaft und Psychoanalyse. Eine Einführung*. 1972. Reprint, Stuttgart: Reclam 2001.

Whyte, Lancelot Law. *The Unconscious Before Freud*. With a foreword by Edith Sitwell. London: Tavistock, 1962.

Williams, Linda Ruth. *Critical Desire: Psychoanalysis and the Literary Subject*. London: Edward Arnold, 1995.

Wittgenstein, Ludwig. *Lectures & Conversations on Aesthetics, Psychology and Religion*. Ed. Cyril Barrett. Compiled from notes taken by Yorick Smythies, Rush Rhees, and James Taylor. Oxford: Blackwell, 1966.

Wolff, Reinhold, ed. *Psychoanalytische Literaturwissenschaft*. Munich: Fink, 1975.

Wollheim, Richard. *Freud*. 2nd ed. London: Fontana, 1991.

Wright, Elizabeth. "Modern Psychoanalytic Criticism." In *Modern Literary Theory: A Comparative Introduction*, ed. Ann Jefferson and David Robey, 145–65. 2nd ed. London: Batsford, 1986.

———. *Psychoanalytic Criticism: Theory in Practice*. 1984. Reprint, London: Routledge, 1993.

Index